# Studies in Big Data

Volume 120

The series "Studies in Big Data" (SBD) publishes new developments and advances in the various areas of Big Data- quickly and with a high quality. The intent is to cover the theory, research, development, and applications of Big Data, as embedded in the fields of engineering, computer science, physics, economics and life sciences. The books of the series refer to the analysis and understanding of large, complex, and/or distributed data sets generated from recent digital sources coming from sensors or other physical instruments as well as simulations, crowd sourcing, social networks or other internet transactions, such as emails or video click streams and other. The series contains monographs, lecture notes and edited volumes in Big Data spanning the areas of computational intelligence including neural networks, evolutionary computation, soft computing, fuzzy systems, as well as artificial intelligence, data mining, modern statistics and Operations research, as well as self-organizing systems. Of particular value to both the contributors and the readership are the short publication timeframe and the world-wide distribution, which enable both wide and rapid dissemination of research output.

The books of this series are reviewed in a single blind peer review process.

Indexed by SCOPUS, EI Compendex, SCIMAGO and zbMATH.

All books published in the series are submitted for consideration in Web of Science.

Sofia Scataglini · Silvia Imbesi · Gonçalo Marques
Editors

# mHealth and Human-Centered Design Towards Enhanced Health, Care, and Well-being

Springer

*Editors*
Sofia Scataglini
Faculty of Medicine and Health Sciences
Department of Rehabilitation Sciences
and Physiotherapy, Center for Health
and Technology (CHaT), 4D4ALL Lab
University of Antwerp
Antwerpen, Belgium

Silvia Imbesi
Dipartimento di Architettura
Università degli Studi di Ferrara
Ferrara, Italy

Gonçalo Marques
Department of Science and Technology
Polytechnic Institute of Coimbra
Technology and Management School
of Oliveira do Hospital
Oliveira do Hospital, Portugal

ISSN 2197-6503 ISSN 2197-6511 (electronic)
Studies in Big Data
ISBN 978-981-99-3988-6 ISBN 978-981-99-3989-3 (eBook)
https://doi.org/10.1007/978-981-99-3989-3



This Springer imprint is published by the registered company Springer Nature Singapore Pte Ltd.
The registered company address is: 152 Beach Road, #21-01/04 Gateway East, Singapore 189721, Singapore

# Preface

The book explores the current state of Human-Centered Design (HCD) applied to mHealth projects from the perspective of users' health, care, and well-being. New opportunities for developing specific solutions aiming at enhancing living conditions have been opened up by the current increase of interest in improving people's quality of life thanks to innovative approaches related to a different conception of prevention, care, and cure. Nowadays research organizations, stakeholders, and academia can take advantage of innovative approaches to support the current changes in society and people's necessities. Moreover, opportunities provided by recent mHeatlh technologies allow the design of products, services, systems, and processes created to empower the well-being of people they are addressed to, considering specifically their needs and the ones of people taking care of them.

This volume describes the state of the art of mHealth systems conceived to support several specific categories of users in monitoring their health conditions and adopting healthy daily behaviors.

Furthermore, this volume introduces updates about new technologies: mHealth, eHealth, telemedicine and telehealth, IoT applications, wearables for pervasive and tailored healthcare, common input devices, robotics, and others. In addition, the topics are examined in their current applications in several research fields, such as wearable devices, smart living environments, activity recognition tools, and virtual care assistance. All these different perspectives have in common the application of HCD methodologies for the definition of objectives and strategies to effectively fulfil users' requirements.

The offered framework of relevant applications and projects has been proposed by international teams of professors, researchers, and professionals applying their different backgrounds in the field of innovative healthcare.

This book includes 11 chapters focusing on relevant topics for enhanced health, care, and well-being.

In Chapter "Involving End Users in Risk-Based Co-design", the authors analyze technologies that could impact the adoption of mHealth devices and how to leverage co-design strategies that could be used to improve the adoption and usability of mHealth solutions.

Chapter "Phygital Mental Health: Opportunities and Challenges" focuses on potential applications of this paradigm to mental health, with special attention to the mHealth solutions dedicated to monitoring and improving the psychological well-being of people navigating across physical and digital worlds.

Chapter "Data Uncertainty and m-Health Interaction Design for Aging People" focuses on the experiential nature of the interaction with digital technology for the aging population. In particular, the chapter discusses wearable technologies from a variety of perspectives, ranging from quality of interaction and user experience to data and information provision.

Chapter "Digital Twins and Healthcare: Quick Overview and Human-Centric Perspectives" presents introductory perspectives on Digital Twins and Healthcare as an overview of opportunities and critical aspects that must be handled to fully benefit from these novel technological solutions even before their actual development and access to the market.

Chapter "mHealth for Well-Being: Case Studies in Physiological, Cognitive, and Affective Sensing" presents two mHealth case studies: a mobile stress management solution and a mobile- and wearable-based cognitive analysis solution but also discusses key concerns/challenges in creating mHealth solutions for mental health and well-being.

Chapter "Design Considerations of Mobile Applications for Healthy Living" comprises important information about mobile health applications, their main challenges, and specifics of the research to define design considerations for this kind of applications.

Chapter "Evaluation Review of Mobile Apps Supporting Adolescents' and Young Adults' Mental Health" analyzes the existing mental health apps for adolescents and young adults which are explored and assessed by utilizing the Evaluation Model Screener which is a part of the American Psychiatric Association Comprehensive App Evaluation Model.

Chapter "An Overview of the Effects of Music on Tourette Syndrome" provides an overview of the beneficial relationship between music, musicians, and Tourette syndrome.

Chapter "Artificial Intelligence Applications and Social Assistive Robotics to Counteract Cognitive Decline in the Older Population: Evidence from Trials in Real Settings" aims to update the knowledge on the efficacy and applicability of social robotics in the context of supporting a cognitive decline in the older population, from prevention and self-management of initial cognitive impairments to the most advanced phases of dementia.

Chapter "Human-Centered Design to Enhance the Holter Monitor Experience for Elderly People" investigates the Human-Centered Design approach in the specific case of the design of the Holter monitor device for elderly people and illustrates all the phases involved in the research project.

Chapter "Exploring a Configurable Virtual Environment for the Assessment and Diagnosis of the Driver's Psychophysical State" describes the development and validation of a configurable and scalable virtual environment, conceived to help researchers to set up the environment freely according to their research needs.

Academics, designers, engineers, and healthcare professionals who aim to encourage collaboration between academia, stakeholders, and research institutions are the target audience of this book.

On this occasion, we would like to recognize the authors, reviews, and book managers who collaborated to make this publication possible. Your professionalism, enthusiasm, and passion allowed this project to be accomplished. We hope that this book can continue to inspire academics, entrepreneurs, stakeholders, and research organizations to support educational innovation.

Antwerp, Belgium — Sofia Scataglini
Ferrara, Italy — Silvia Imbesi
Oliveira do Hospital, Coimbra, Portugal — Gonçalo Marques

# Contents

# About the Editors

**Sofia Scataglini** is a Biomedical Engineer and Visiting Professor at Antwerp University in the Faculty of Medicine and Health Sciences, Department of Rehabilitation Sciences and Physiotherapy, Antwerp, Belgium. Prof. Sofia Scataglini is recognized with the title of European Ergonomist (Eur. Erg.), CREE. In doing so, she is a member of the Scientific Committee of the International Ergonomics Association (IEA) and Chair of the IEA Technical Committee on Digital Human Modeling and Simulation. Sofia is the founder of the Digital Human Modeling by Women group (DHMW), which is dedicated to promoting women in STEAM around the world. Sofia organizes congresses related to applied human factors, ergonomics, wearables, and digital human modeling (DHM). She is involved in different TC groups for standardization, such as at the national (NBN), European (CENELEC), and international levels (ISO and IEC) for ergonomics, biomechanics, wearables, smart textiles, PPE, and clothing. She is also an active editor, writer, and reviewer of books and journals and scientific grants focusing on sensors, medicine, health and care, modeling and simulation, standardization, ergonomics, biomechanics, and design. Her research activities focus on the research and design of products, systems, environments, and services for the health, care, and well-being of people using co-design and user-centered design methods combined with ergonomics.

**Silvia Imbesi** is Architect and Industrial Designer. Currently, she works as Research Fellow in Inclusive Design at the Department of Architecture of the University of Ferrara, Italy. She is an expert in user-centered methodologies for the design of products, services, and systems. She uses to develop design projects for niche users belonging to fragile categories, particularly in healthcare devices related to the Internet of Things. Since 2009, Silvia Imbesi has worked as Freelance Architect and Designer, collaborating with other professionals, companies, industries, and institutions for the development of projects and design research. Starting in 2012, she collaborated with the University of Ferrara as Contract Professor and participated in several kinds of research related to user-centered methodologies and inclusive devices related to the Internet of Things, innovative teaching methods, etc. Silvia

Imbesi authored many international publications about Human-Centered Design, inclusive design, the Internet of Things, wearable devices, human factors, mHealth systems, data visualization, etc.

**Gonçalo Marques** holds a Ph.D. in Computer Science Engineering and is Senior member of the Portuguese Engineering Association (Ordem dos Engenheiros). He is currently working as Assistant Professor lecturing courses on programming, multimedia, and database systems. Furthermore, he worked as a Software Engineer in the Innovation and Development unit of Groupe PSA automotive industry from 2016 to 2017 and in the IBM group from 2018 to 2019. His current research interests include the Internet of Things, Enhanced Living Environments, machine learning, e-health, telemedicine, medical and healthcare systems, indoor air quality monitoring and assessment, and wireless sensor networks. He has more than 80 publications in international journals and conferences, is a frequent reviewer of journals and international conferences and is also involved in several edited books projects.

# Involving End Users in Risk-Based Co-design

**Federico Sternini, Giacinto Barresi, and Alice Ravizza**

## 1 Introduction

Among all opportunities provided in the field of healthcare by recent innovative digital technologies, the increased availability of mobile and digital solutions can improve the effectiveness of complex health programs, either public or private. The technological development of such solutions led the policymakers and the public institutions to identify a regulatory framework suitable for the safe and effective development of new products that could allow the users and the patients to obtain a net increase in the quality of life or care. Currently, the European Union introduced major regulations providing manufacturers and research groups not only constraints but also opportunities for the development of new digital solutions in the healthcare field. The core regulations are the General Data Protection Regulation (GDPR), which aims to protect European citizens while ensuring an adequate standard for the management and circulation of personal data, and the twin Medical Device Regulation (MDR) and In Vitro Medical Device Regulation (IVDR), which introduced Europe to a universal regulatory framework that includes evaluation and special considerations on medical device software, a sector of the medical device field that gained so much importance to obtain a specific classification rule [1–3]. The special consideration of

F. Sternini (✉) · A. Ravizza
USE-ME-D srl, I3P Politecnico di Torino, Torino, Italy
e-mail: federico.sternini@polito.it

A. Ravizza
e-mail: ing.ravizza@gmail.com

F. Sternini
PolitoBIOMed Lab, Politecnico di Torino, Torino, Italy

G. Barresi
Rehab Technologies Lab, Istituto Italiano di Tecnologia (IIT), Genoa, Italy
e-mail: giacinto.barresi@iit.it



S. Scataglini et al. (eds.), *mHealth and Human-Centered Design Towards Enhanced Health, Care, and Well-Being*, Studies in Big Data 120,
https://doi.org/10.1007/978-981-99-3989-3_1

software in the regulations and its application across Europe is intended to level the certification process for all manufacturers, and therefore ensure increased distribution and availability of safe, controlled and high-quality products, furthering the digital transformation that is running in Europe.

The technological evolution to digitalization allows shifting the focus from the traditional approach of finding the best treatment suitable for many patients to an innovative approach that seeks the personalised, optimal management of the whole clinical process for each patient. In this context, this chapter aims to propose an approach and a set of techniques for the involvement of end-users in the design phase without affecting the safety of the medical device. The chapter will first analyze the new technological features introduced by the last introduced medical device category, i.e. Digital Therapeutics, their challenges and chances for the patient-centred design.

In what follows, the authors then analyzed the technologies that could impact the adoption of m-Health devices and how to leverage the co-design strategies that could be used to improve the adoption and usability of m-Health solutions. The proposed approach is based on the experience of the authors in the medical device industry and the co-design field, keeping as reference international safety and efficacy standards. In this chapter the authors tried to identify strategies, methodologies and boundaries to involve end-users in the design process of medical devices using as the main target and reference the risk profile of the newly designed devices (that should not be negatively affected), to foster innovation and the involvement of end-users not only in the research field but even in the industrial context.

## 2 A New Approach to Integrated Care Pathways

In the past, the approach to definition and validation of integrated care pathways has been based on literature review, critical appraisal, multidisciplinary consultation, and grading of recommendations using as reference the level of evidence [4]. In this approach, the patient was idealized as a "standard" or "most common" patient to allow the classification of the various integrated care pathway, reflecting the patient's main characteristics [5]. On the other hand, personalized management of each integrated care pathway may lead to improved efficacy in the clinical impact, improved efficiency in the use of resources and eventually to a more equitable distribution of health resources.

A personalized approach to the integrated care pathway may be strongly supported by technological solutions in the field of Digital therapeutics (DTx). While a complete consensus on the meaning of DTx is not yet reached in the scientific community, the best definition of DTx can be "*Digital therapeutics (DTx) deliver evidence-based therapeutic interventions that are driven by high-quality software programs to prevent, manage, or treat a medical disorder or disease*" [6].

To provide useful means for a personalised approach to care, DTx should adopt some specific technical functions. For example, the capability to provide, from a standardized anamnesis questionnaire, specific identification of patient subgroups and a disease pattern recognition may improve the adequate timing of planning of an existing integrated care pathway.

A specific analysis, based on the design suggestions emerged from the experience of the authors and from the interpretation of the best practices proposed by the Digital Therapeutics Alliance [7], of the most common technical features of DTx that may have an impact on the personalization of an integrated care pathway is summarized in Table 1.

The personalized approach hereby presented is a potential solution that leverages the main technologies currently available in the m-Health development field.

## 3 Technologies to Lower the Gap and Foster the Adoption of mHealth Technologies

This target may be reached through the adoption and use of all available mHealth technologies, leveraging the accessibility of mobile solutions for personalised healthcare through easily accessible mobile devices, even in medium- and low-income scenarios. Some accessibility features, both from the technological and the usability point of view, may be taken into consideration when developing a personalised care approach that is intended for different income scenarios, to provide accessible mHealth solutions [8]. The designers should take the opportunity of the customization of the mHealth technology and consider all the available features and know-how and prefer the most impactful approaches to lower economical, educational and digital gaps, as proposed in Table 2.

## 4 Co-design to Foster the Adoption of mHealth Technologies

Co-design is based on the structured involvement of stakeholders in the process of ideation. To maximize the efficiency and repeatability of this involvement, specific techniques for formative activities during usability design should be taken into account. Standard IEC/TR 62366-2 describes several such techniques: amongst those, some techniques are particularly appropriate to co-design of mHealth technologies [9, 10]. The technologies that could result in the most adequate are the ones suitable for the early development stages like the ones that are usually associated with the early formative stage and that can leverage the potential of digital tools [11]. Table 3 presents the identification of the main characteristics that guide the selection of the techniques proposed by the international standard for the planning of the co-design activities of mHealth technologies, as identified by the authors [10]. In Table 3 are included only the techniques that foresee the participation of end-users.

**Table 1** mHealth technical features and their impact

| Technical feature | Description of functionality (example) | Potential impact |
|---|---|---|
| Customisation of versions | Possibility to customise the device in accordance with the user's knowledge and digital literacy (an app for the home follow-up of surgery patients is provided by an onboarding function that assesses the capability of the patient to interpret signs and symptoms of an infection) | The user would have a user interface adequate to its expectations and habits, easing the learning process and minimizing any bias or error that could be introduced by usability pitfalls |
| Interoperability and IoT for hardware medical devices with widespread communication protocols that enable the end-user to choose the best technology | Use of widely adopted interoperation standards like FHIR-HL7 or DICOM (a platform for the long-term management of overweight patients by dieticians is synchronized with the information on the GP database) | The definition of additional standards in emerging fields could allow physicians and patients to not have limited choices regarding medical instrumentation and devices. In addition, the prompt definition of interoperation standards from the first phases of device adoption should allow manufacturers to reduce the development efforts by implementing the proper requirement from the first development phases |
| Identification of patients' subgroups and pattern recognition | Identification of behavioural characteristics concerning the DTx use and subsequent user experience adaptation (an app intended for chronic patients has an onboarding interview that classifies the patient personal approach to his/her chronic condition) | The automated identification of subgroups and behaviours could lead the DTx to better match the needs of each user. In addition, on the other hand, it could allow the DTx to reduce all the elements of the user interface that could interfere with the clinical benefit provision |

(continued)

**Table 1** (continued)

| Technical feature | Description of functionality (example) | Potential impact |
|---|---|---|
| Adaptation of language to the expectations of end-users | Capability to define the language of the user interface through configuration files and the possibility to change it in accordance with nationality and educational background | The professional user could use the device with a technical language that is most adequate for the management of the clinical path, while on the other hand, the patient would use the user interface with terms that are adequate to their educational level, without feeling neither paternalised nor overwhelmed |
| Approach to involvement: responsibilization, patient empowerment or gamification depending on the patient preference | Different functions that customise the involvement of each different end user (for end users that prefer a traditional interaction: possibility for the patient to request a physician telemedicine visit through the app calendar) (for end users that prefer gamification: trophies) | The inclusion of patient empowerment that is most suitable to the patient character could allow an increased self-awareness and responsibilities for therapy self-management, leading to increased adherence and producing more reliable and significant data to be analyzed by the physician |

**Table 2** Proposed heuristic principles for an equitable approach to personalized DTx

| Heuristic principle | Expected outcome | Technological solution |
|---|---|---|
| Bridging the technological gap | Provision of DTX across different income settings | Provision of apps that are adequately designed to be installed in legacy versions of operative systems<br>Provision of apps with low computational power<br>Maintenance of apps versions compliant with legacy versions of operative systems over time<br>Compatibility with low-income dedicated operative systems<br>Long-term support to allow proper use in second-hand devices |
| Bridging the educational gap | Provision of DTx across different educational levels | Simplified language<br>Provision of in-app tools for tailored educational contents |
| Bridging the digital gap | Provision of DTx across different age groups | Availability of a simplified interface for users with low digital literacy<br>Provision of in-app shortcuts to the most impactful patient interactions |

**Table 3** IEC 62366 methods and their characteristics

| Method as per Table E.1 of IEC 62366–2:2016 | Adequate to SaMDs | Need to involve experts | Need to involve end-users | Usability evaluation phase |
|---|---|---|---|---|
| FMEA and FTA | Yes | No | Yes | Late formative |
| Observation | No | No | Yes | Early formative |
| One-on-one interviews | Yes | No | Yes | Early formative |
| Participatory design | Yes | Yes | Yes | Late formative |
| PCA analysis | Yes | Yes | Yes | Late formative |
| Simulation | Yes | Yes | Yes | Late formative and summative |
| Surveys | No | No | Yes | Late formative and summative |
| Task analysis | Yes | Yes | Yes | Late formative and summative |
| Time-and-motion studies | Maybe | No | Yes | Late formative and summative |
| Usability tests | Yes | Yes | Yes | Late formative and summative |
| Workload assessment | No | No | Yes | Late formative and summative |

## *4.1 Patient Engagement*

It is already widely accepted that the role of patients in this shift will be the core: patients are more and more actively involved in the management of their healthcare journey, thanks to more pervasive medical devices and technologies such as smart health solutions and mHealth devices. Amongst the different heuristics, some are more intuitive and may be presented to the non-technical co-designers while others require a more structured approach by the technical co-designers.

Before presenting these heuristics (subsection 4.3) it is necessary to highlight how any strategy to co-design health technologies must be based on methodologies that need to bring the attention of the potential final users towards devices that could appear useless and intrusive, especially when they are still at prototype stage [12, 13]. Accordingly, a primary barrier to the patient's engagement can be technology acceptance, which can affect the co-design process itself. Overall, Technology Acceptance Models are typically enriched with new dimensions when we consider specific types of applications, like games, considering their perceived usefulness and usability, alongside the age, gender, and culture of the users) [14]. Interestingly, the growing confidence of ageing cohorts in handling mobile devices will affect their acceptance. Beyond the compulsory premise of technology acceptance, Lavallee et al. stated how the importance of patient engagement is underestimated in most investigations, even if it could lead to major improvements in product design and development [15].

In particular, the Lavallee et al. discussed the conditions to engage patients in the co-design of mobile health tools for the surveillance of surgical site infections [15]. The authors highlighted how the healthcare industry can take advantage of patient-owned devices like smartphones and tablets to monitor data for postoperative management. Thus, mHealth can exploit mobile systems as familiar devices to gather data on users' behaviours and needs, a fundamental premise for any user-centred design procedure. Furthermore, the involvement of the final users in activities like workshops can promote a self-care attitude and a higher clinical adherence of the patients.

Triggering a creative mindset in activities for mHealth co-design depends on pondering the corpus of knowledge on motivation and engagement in interactive systems [16]. This is the key for proposing approaches able to catch the users beyond traditional workshops. An example of innovation in this field is constituted by the IoT Un-Kit Experience: a set of components (e.g., sensors, actuators) that are presented to older people as uncompleted and decontextualized [17]. However, the participants in a co-design session are invited to explore and create IoT systems through these items to obtain meaningful solutions from their point of view. This way, the user-centred designer can collect the users' feedback by keeping them involved through an autonomous creative process.

Furthermore, literature also proposed to carry the iterative and participatory design processes beyond the release of the product itself. Indeed, through appropriate sensors, it is possible to gather information on the use of the device by engaging its users through approaches of continuous co-design and designing-in-use [18]. Summing up, the engagement of patients in co-design can occur during the process itself or after it as well, according to the data that can be collected after the product release.

## *4.2 Physician Engagement*

Specialised healthcare professionals are gaining an active part in the use, customisation and management of mHealth technologies that reshape traditional clinical practice [19]. Involvement of experts of the clinical field, such as example physicians, may be fostered by guided focus groups in which a small panel of experts is first guided through the use experience, for example by a cognitive walkthrough, and then participates in an open discussion on the general aspects of safety and efficiency of the eHealth technology. In such open discussions, the physicians' expectations in terms of the quantity of information and the kind of presentation of the information may be determined. Some structured discussion, guided by a focus group coordinator, may be obtained by posing product-specific questions, based on heuristic principles [20, 21].

For example, for the heuristic "consistency and standards" a device-specific question may be posed as "*Is the device interface consistent with other devices commonly used for this clinical application*?" Or, for example, for the heuristic "help and documentation", a device-specific question may be posed as "Is the language used in the information for use clear and clinically appropriate?".

Another technique for structured discussion is based firstly on the determination of the device's testable technical requirements and then on posing questions intended to determine if the testable technical requirement has been met by the mHealth technology, a technique already proven effective for the evaluation of SaMDs usability evaluation [21]. A practical example of this procedure can be described using as reference the development and usability assessment process implemented in the realization of a software as a medical device for intraoperative surgical planning [22]. The software is based on a touchless user interface, realized by sensing the hands of the user in the sensing volume and providing the user with a set of gestures for the management of the visualization of the 3D model of the target organ. One of the analyzed testable technical requirements was associated with organ model management ("*The hand gestures and the menu setting shall allow to isolate and change the transparency of the parts belonging to organ model in an intuitive manner*"). First, a Focus Group was completed, and after the completion of the focus group, the users were asked to fill out a questionnaire intended to evaluate the testable technical requirements. From the results of the questionnaire, the designers investigated the root causes of the main usability issues that affected the testable requirements and proposed an improvement for further iteration of the development of the device. Finally, in the summative phase, a net improvement in the evaluation of the testable technical requirement was observed.

## *4.3 How to Involve Users*

There is a need to involve patients and clinical professionals as an active part not only in the management but also in the design stage of the health journey. An early-stage involvement allows the actors of the healthcare process to provide designers with their impressions, needs and goals. A new approach for the design of new services as in mHealth is required. Such an approach should include patients and professional end-users of technologies as main actors not only in the day-by-day use but also in the ideation and development of such technologies.

Table 4 uses as a reference the Nielsen Heuristics and presents the proposal of the authors for the management of different aspects of co-design participation, based on the level of professional knowledge of the co-designers. This proposal has been applied to the improvements or developments of software as a Medical Device, but in future, it will be hopefully adopted from the first iterations of the design of many medical devices. Additionally, future works could adopt this approach in synergy with others already explored in literature [23–25].

**Table 4** Co-design aspects based on the Nielsen heuristics [26]

| Heuristic | Involvement of co-designers | Standardised technique |
|---|---|---|
| Visibility<br>*#1: Visibility of system status*<br>*The design should always keep users informed about what is going on, through appropriate feedback within a reasonable amount of time* | An open approach for the determination of the specific system status is recommended. Examples include current step of the clinical procedure and the current patient | Use of walkthrough in preliminary iterations<br>Simulation in further iterations<br>Guided application of ETA[a] in case the system is not visible |
| Match<br>*#2: Match between system and the real world*<br>*The design should speak the users' language. Use words, phrases, and concepts familiar to the user, rather than internal jargon. Follow real-world conventions, making information appear in a natural and logical order* | For both professional and non-professional co-designers, the involvement should be based on the verification:<br>• that the mHealth technology is consistent with their general expectations on the meaning of icons, symbols and other interface connectors<br>• that the language used in the interface is clear to the reader, clinically correct, and respectful | Use of sketches or simulations<br>Guided application of ETA in case the information is misinterpreted |
| Control<br>*#3: User control and freedom*<br>*Users often perform actions by mistake. They need a clearly marked "emergency exit" to leave the unwanted action without having to go through an extended process* | For both professional and non-professional co-designers, the involvement should be based on the creation of use paths that then allow defining where to provide the "emergency exit" and where, on the other hand, require a formal saving of data before the possibility of leaving the interface page | Focus groups based on the review of the visual representation of the use path (for example as a flow chart), the guided definition of the steps in which the user shall save the inputted data before leaving the interface page |
| Consistency<br>*#4: Consistency and standards*<br>*Users should not have to wonder whether different words, situations, or actions mean the same thing. Follow platform and industry conventions* | Standards in the medical device industry are very complex and strict<br>For professional co-designers, such for example physicians or nurses, the involvement should be based on the verification that the mHealth technology is consistent with the general clinical guidelines<br>Additionally, specific technical activity for the consistency of the interface with standardized symbols should be conducted by regulatory professionals | Checklist for compliance with clinical guidelines<br>Checklist for compliance to regulatory requirements, for example, application of MDR, Annex I clause 23 and application of ISO 20417 [2, 28] |

(continued)

**Table 4** (continued)

| Heuristic | Involvement of co-designers | Standardised technique |
|---|---|---|
| Error prevention<br>*#5: Error prevention*<br>*Good error messages are important, but the best designs carefully prevent problems from occurring in the first place. Either eliminate error-prone conditions or check for them and present users with a confirmation option before they commit to the action* | In the medical device field, use errors may lead to clinical risk. Error prevention shall be preferably addressed by safe-by-design solutions<br>Both professional and non-professional co-designers should be involved in the ideation of the error-prevention features and, even more importantly, in the validation of the effectiveness of such measures | Use of walkthrough in preliminary iterations<br>Simulation in further iterations |
| Memory<br>*#6: Recognition rather than recall*<br>*Minimize the user's memory load by making elements, actions, and options visible. The user should not have to remember information from one part of the interface to another. Information required to use the design (e.g. field labels or menu items) should be visible or easily retrievable when needed* | For both professional and non-professional co-designers, the involvement should be based on the minimisation of information to be memorized from one screen to be used in the next one<br>For non-professional co-designers, this is particularly valid for acronyms, technical words and clinical lingo<br>On the other hand, professional co-designers typically remember specific terms and information that may not need to be repeated in the interface | Checklist for compliance with clinical guidelines<br>Formal review of the quantity of information for each interface screen<br>Focus groups<br>Dedicated user testing for non-professional users, involving representatives of users with different levels of education |
| Flexibility<br>*#7: Flexibility and efficiency of use*<br>*Shortcuts—hidden from novice users—may speed up the interaction for the expert user such that the design can cater to both inexperienced and experienced users. Allow users to tailor frequent actions* | For both professional and non-professional co-designers, the involvement should be based on the creation of use paths that may then guide the definition of pre-defined shortcuts | Focus groups based on the review of the visual representation of the use path (for example as a flow chart), the guided definition of shortcuts in the path |

(continued)

**Table 4** (continued)

| Heuristic | Involvement of co-designers | Standardised technique |
|---|---|---|
| Minimalist<br>#8: *Aesthetic and minimalist design*<br>*Interfaces should not contain information which is irrelevant or rarely needed. Every extra unit of information in an interface competes with the relevant units of information and diminishes their relative visibility* | For non-professional co-designers, the involvement should be based on the request to define, according to their opinions and expertise, which information shall always be present on all the screens of the interface and which information is redundant or confusing<br>As a general example, non-professional users prefer to have the unit of measure of any measurement already defined by the interface and consistent with the local habits (this is particularly interesting for the units of measure for body weight)<br>For professional co-designers the requirement is similar but there is a specific requirement that the minimal information presented is consistent with the guidelines regarding human error prevention in medicine. For example, the patient's name or code shall always be present and clearly visible | Checklist for compliance with clinical guidelines<br>Formal review of the quantity of information for each interface screen<br>Focus groups |
| Error messages<br>#9: *Help users recognize, diagnose, and recover from errors*<br>*Error messages should be expressed in plain language (no error codes), precisely indicate the problem, and constructively suggest a solution* | For both professional and non-professional co-designers, the involvement should be based on the verification that the error messages are perceivable and clear to the reader, clinically correct, and respectful<br>Similarly, the proposed solution/remediation to the error should be clear | Checklist for compliance with clinical guidelines<br>Checklist for compliance to regulatory requirements, for example, application of MDR, Annex I clause 23 and application of ISO 20417 [2, 28] |

(continued)

In any case, the patients and the physicians do have particular information and needs that should be satisfied but could lack an adequate background regarding the techniques for development and the design of devices that could have an impact on patient and operator's health. Therefore, for each one of those involved in the design stage technique, an adequate policy should be defined to preserve the safety of the device and to ensure adequate repeatability of the medical device design stage.

**Table 4** (continued)

| Heuristic | Involvement of co-designers | Standardised technique |
|---|---|---|
| Documentation<br>*#10: Help and documentation*<br>*It's best if the system doesn't need any additional explanation. However, it may be necessary to provide documentation to help users understand how to complete their tasks* | The information provided in writing should be capable to support the use and understanding of residual risks<br>For both professional and non-professional co-designers, the involvement should be based on the verification that the documentation is perceivable (readable, audible and so on), clear, and complete | Checklist for compliance with clinical guidelines<br>Checklist for compliance to regulatory requirements, for example, application of MDR, Annex I clause 23 and application of ISO 20417 [2, 28] |

[a]Event Tree Analysis: ETA is a causal analytical technique that is based on an analysis of a sequence of actions and events that can lead to a negative outcome [27]

The following tables summarize the main components of a medical device and a medical device user interface with a proposal related to the specific aspect of the management of that medical device aspect, highlighting the roles and the responsibilities that can be managed by the different stakeholders. Table 5 proposes detailed policies for the management of all the heuristics identified by Zhang et al., while Table 6 focuses on all the relevant components that should be planned and defined for regulatory and safety purposes [20].

## 5 Impact of Co-design

The application of the techniques and processes described in the previous sections could affect the design and development of medical technologies. Nevertheless, the proposed approach should not compromise the safety and reliability of the design and development process. Traditionally, designers are required to implement risk mitigation measures in their technology, with an a priori definition of the risk control measures and subsequently verifying their effectiveness, while in some of the proposed techniques, end-users are included in the process that identifies and implement the risk control measures. This approach should ensure a higher success rate and greater efficacy of the risk control measure. The techniques and policies defined in the previous sections should ensure an adequate procedure for the identification of the main actors for each activity that is involved in the design and development process, thus reducing the chances of introducing additional risks and increasing the chances of a successful proposal of technical solutions. The designers should put in place a rigorous application of a reliable risk management procedure and risk control measure verification, in accordance with ISO 14971 requirements [30].

**Table 5** Policy for co-design approach on each aspect that characterizes the medical device focused on the user interface

| Aspect | Policy |
|---|---|
| Consistency<br>*Consistency and standards. Users should not have to wonder whether different words, situations, or actions mean the same thing. Standards and conventions in product design should be followed* | During the design of the user interface, the proposed approach is to present a mockup to patients and physicians in the early development stage of the device, to avoid big differences with the tools and devices usually used by both user groups. During the later development stages, an iterative approach with different short sessions related to portions of the device should be presented to the patients, so that they can confirm all the user interfaces. Professional users instead could be more active in the design phase not only evaluating the mockups but also providing guidelines and approaches used in the common clinical practice |
| Visibility<br>*Visibility of system state. Users should be informed about what is going on with the system through appropriate feedback and display of information* | The designers should identify the set of information that the device should present to users for safety reasons, including aspects related to information for safe use, advertences on non-eliminable risks, and regulatory requirements such as specific symbols. The end-users should be included in the design activities for the identification of the most appropriate way to present the information and to suggest presenting additional data that is not directly related to the device safety but that can be impactful on the device user experience |
| Match<br>*Match between system and world. The image of the system perceived by users should match the model the users have about the system* | Before the beginning of the user interface design activity, the end-users should be invited to discuss the device's intended use and the device's potential user experience. An adequate technique may be a cognitive walk-through. The involvement in this phase should allow designers, patients and physicians to identify any device (either similar or not to the device under development) that can have set expectations in the user regarding some user interfaces or user experiences. The designers should take note of these devices and identify with the end-users which are the components that could set the expectations for the user |
| Minimalist<br>*Minimalist. Any extraneous information is a distraction and a slow-down* | The process should be the same as the Visibility aspect. In addition, the users should evaluate how much the requested information may be redundant or confounding<br>A specific focus group may be held for alarms and notifications, to assess any possible alarm overload to end-users due to multiple notifications and alarms<br>In addition, a risk evaluation method such as an ETA may be used to define a policy for the criticality of alarms and notifications. For example, a critical alarm may appear as a pop-up in the centre of the interface and may only be solved by a user action. On the other hand, a non-critical notification may appear as a sidebar and automatically disappear after some seconds |

(continued)

**Table 5** (continued)

| Aspect | Policy |
|---|---|
| Memory *Minimize memory load. Users should not be required to memorize a lot of information to carry out tasks. Memory load reduces users' capacity to carry out the main tasks* | The designers should identify, using as a reference all the devices obtained for the management of the Match aspect, and all design features that allow the user to reduce the use of memory. In addition, experience from devices of different purposes can be included (e.g. autocomplete inspired by smartphone keyboards) and ask end-users if the newly suggested features may be considered useful<br>An adequate approach may be the identification of main device tasks and then a function analysis, to determine what should be the automated actions and what actions should be initiated by the end-user |
| Feedback *Informative feedback. Users should be given prompt and informative feedback about their actions* | The suggested approach is similar to the one proposed for the management of the consistency aspect. During the first phase in the early stage of development, the designers should ask end-users to identify the main feedbacks that should be presented by the device. In later stages of development, the end-users may evaluate the proposed feedback. For example, in a clinical data edit phase, the user would like to receive a confirmation of the correct and complete edit from the interface, by the means of a pop-up, "all edits are saved" raised after the data saving |
| Flexibility *Flexibility and efficiency. Users always learn and users are always different. Give users the flexibility of creating customization and shortcuts to accelerate their performance* | The designers should propose a user experience suitable for standard users. Nevertheless, the inclusion of the users in the co-design stage in various iterations should be used to give chances for users that are already proficient to propose shortcuts and alternate paths for the management of the use flow. This should be eased by the designers by asking the end-users which parts of the user interface they find most annoying and pointlessly time-consuming |
| Message *Good error messages. The messages should be informative enough such that users can understand the nature of errors, learn from errors, and recover from errors* | The designers should propose to end-users the conditions and situations that should be notified to users as identified during the risk analysis phase. The end users then should actively propose the best way to communicate the warnings and the notifications to be most effective. In addition, the end-users should describe the most effective way to communicate to users in case of technical errors, including which level of actions can be asked to end-users from a notification/error message |

(continued)

The approach exploits the opportunities given by the current European Regulation on medical devices and the related international standards. Here we recall that the European Regulations define a set of General Performance and Safety Requirements (GSPR) that each medical device shall satisfy. The provision of such requirements is intended to define a safety level adequate to all users and patients while fostering innovation, leaving room for innovative technologies and design processes to be introduced [2]. The regulators are aware that a "no risk" level is not achievable for

**Table 5** (continued)

| Aspect | Policy |
|---|---|
| Error<br>*Prevent errors. It is always better to design interfaces that prevent errors from happening in the first place* | The proposed approach is the full application of the IEC 62366 workflow to the user interface evaluation, including the inclusion of a formative evaluation from the first design stages and repeating it iteratively until a significant prototype of the user interface is obtained Specific walkthroughs may be held to determine the adequate path for error correction. Particular attention may be deemed to data insertion interfaces and redundant information, understanding which automated controls are considered not excessively invasive by the users. For example, the interface may suggest automatically data previously saved or complete consistency checks over inserted data (e.g. weight of an adult should not be lower than 10 kg) without being perceived as a complication of the use flow |
| Closure<br>*Clear closure. Every task has a beginning and an end. Users should be clearly notified about the completion of a task* | The proposed approach is the full application of the IEC 62366 workflow to the user interface evaluation, including the inclusion of a formative evaluation from the first design stages and repeating it iteratively until a significant prototype of the user interface is obtained [9, 29] |
| Undo<br>*Reversible actions. Users should be allowed to recover from errors. Reversible actions also encourage exploratory learning* | The proposed approach is the full application of the IEC 62366 workflow to the user interface evaluation, including the inclusion of a formative evaluation from the first design stages and repeating it iteratively until a significant prototype of the user interface is obtained [9, 29] |
| Language<br>*Use users' language. The language should be always presented in a form understandable by the intended users* | The proposed approach is the inclusion of end-users in the co-design of the texts that compose the user interface from the very beginning of the text drafts. First of all the co-design phase should aim to the identification of the most appropriate language register for each user group. In the following stages, the wording and the messages should be co-designed and evaluated with an approach similar to the one presented for the consistency aspect |
| Control<br>*Users in control. Do not give users the impression that they are controlled by the systems* | The proposed approach is to involve from the very beginning of the user interface design the end-users in the co-design activities to understand which tasks they would like to complete starting the actions autonomously and which tasks they want to be triggered automatically by the mHealth solution. In addition, during the design, they should be included iteratively during the formative phase for the management of the autonomy level of the users |
| Document<br>*Help and documentation. Always provide help when needed* | The users should be involved during the formative phase from the early stages, to understand which is the most adequate means for communication with users in terms of support provision |

**Table 6** Policy for co-design approach on each aspect that characterizes the medical device focused on medical device main features

| Aspect | Policy |
|---|---|
| Intended use | The device's intended use should be proposed by the designers to both professional users and lay users. The main contribution of the intended use proposal to the end-users is the definition of the strategy for the management of the intended use and the adequateness of the proposed mHealth solution for the intended use. In particular, the users should provide a significant contribution in terms of the identification of potential faults in the design (e.g. wrong hypotheses regarding the user desiderata or regarding the user that will be using the proposed solution for that intended use) |
| Intended clinical benefit | The designers should discuss from the start of the design stage the intended clinical benefit with the clinicians and with trained patients the expected clinical benefit. The definition of this aspect from the beginning is intended to drive the management of the data within the device and to drive any clinical trial that will be required for regulatory approval of the mHealth solution<br>Claims on clinical benefit shall be measurable and relevant to all stakeholders |
| Outcome measure | The designers should discuss from the start of the design stage the intended clinical benefit with the clinicians and with trained patients the expected clinical benefit. They should also discuss with both clinicians and trained patients how to measure the intended and expected benefit. The definition of this aspect from the beginning is intended to drive the management of the data within the device and to drive the eventual clinical trial that will be required for regulatory approval of the mHealth solution |
| Accessibility of the device | The accessibility of the device and the way it should be made available to end-users is a key aspect to be shared and planned with all end-users from the beginning, to reduce to the minimum the adoption barriers that could be found by end-users |
| Distribution of the device | In a way similar to the one discussed in the previous point, the users should share with the designers the problems related to the access and the distribution of the device and its updates, including technological, digital literacy and training barriers |

any medical device, so the GSPR are drafted to require a risk–benefit profile of each device beneficial to the patient, and that the evidence of such profile shall be provided with real-world data using an evidence-based medicine approach. In this context, the co-design techniques should not introduce potential issues in the regulatory approval phase and ease the collection of real-world data and aid the design of the device with a beneficial risk–benefit profile.

The approach presented in this chapter defines a design process that involves non-technical co-designers safely and effectively in the design and verification phase of new mHealth technologies. The exploited standards, which are used as a reference for the definition of this process, include ISO 14971 for risk management in medical devices, and IEC 62366 for the usability evaluation of medical devices. The overall structure of the process is based on ISO 13485, which defines the processes for the design of a medical device. This integrated approach ensures that all the regulatory inputs, such as safety, standard compliance and design traceability are maintained [9, 29–32].

The co-design activities can thus be included in a design control process like the following one, in compliance with ISO 13485 [31]. Activities impacted by co-design are presented in **bold**:

- **definition of product specifications**
- **preliminary risk assessment**
- **ideation phase for the preliminary prototype, including the identification of safe-by-design measures**
- manufacturing at laboratory-scale of the preliminary prototype
- **formative testing for the verification of the safe-by-design measures and the proposal of improvements**
- **ideation phase for the advanced prototype, including the upgrades identified in the previous steps**
- manufacturing in pilot scale of the advanced prototype
- **formative testing for the confirmation of the core technical features of the advanced prototype: such tests may be performed in laboratory or by simulation and should include the participation of healthy volunteers**
- **validation for safety, usability and technical performance**
- pre-clinical validation, where possible with the use of a simulated environment
- clinical validation with the involvement of patients in a clinical trial

## 6 Conclusion

The approach to design that will is presented in this chapter is based on the following core aspects:

- **Risk-based approach**: the risk-based approach, clearly described in Annex I of MDR and in ISO 14971, accepts the fact that there is no such thing as a zero-risk device, and requires designers to identify, implement and validate risk control measures with an approach described as "as-low-as-possible" [2, 30]. Therefore, all risk mitigation measures that are technically feasible and effective in reducing the risk, shall be integrated into the device.
- **Identification of user needs**: the identification of user needs targets mostly the clinical needs but also includes needs for education/training and usability. Specific requirements for collecting and reviewing user needs as part of the design input definition are found in ISO 13485 [31].
- **Co-design of the device user interface with stakeholders**: specific techniques for the ideation step can be found in the standard IEC 62366; ideation is typically an iterative process and therefore the complexity of techniques may be chosen according to the evolutive steps [9, 29].

- **Participation of the stakeholders in verification and validation**: specific techniques for the validation step can be found in the standard IEC 62366, but the validation step shall be also integrated with the requirements from ISO 13485 whereas clinical validation requires the collection of clinical data [9, 29, 31].

These four core steps will allow the structuring of a design control process in compliance with the main biomedical standard for quality management systems in the biomedical industry, including IEC 62366 for usability, ISO 13485 for quality management of the design process, ISO 14971 for product risk management [9, 29–31].

## References


1. Regulation (EU) 2016/679 of the European Parliament and of the Council of 27 April 2016 on the protection of natural persons with regard to the processing of personal data and on the free movement of such data, and repealing Directive 95/46/EC (General Data Protection Regulation) (Text with EEA relevance) (2016). Accessed 17 May 2022. http://data.europa.eu/eli/reg/2016/679/2016-05-04/eng
2. Regulation (EU) 2017/745 of the European Parliament and of the Council of 5 April 2017 on medical devices, amending Directive 2001/83/EC, Regulation (EC) No 178/2002 and Regulation (EC) No 1223/2009 and repealing Council Directives 90/385/EEC and 93/42/EEC (Text with EEA relevance)Text with EEA relevance (2020). Accessed 17 May 2022. http://data.europa.eu/eli/reg/2017/745/2020-04-24/eng
3. Regulation (EU) 2017/746 of the European Parliament and of the Council of 5 April 2017 on in vitro diagnostic medical devices and repealing Directive 98/79/EC and Commission Decision 2010/227/EU (Text with EEA relevance)Text with EEA relevance (2022). Accessed 06 Jun 2022. http://data.europa.eu/eli/reg/2017/746/2022-01-28/eng
4. Campbell, H., Hotchkiss, R., Bradshaw, N., Porteous, M.: Integrated care pathways. BMJ **316**(7125), 133–137 (1998)
5. Goldberger, J.J., Buxton, A.E.: Personalized medicine vs guideline-based medicine. JAMA **309**(24), 2559–2560 (2013). https://doi.org/10.1001/jama.2013.6629
6. Digital Therapeutics Alliance, 'Digital Therapeutics—Definition and Core Principles'. November (2019). Accessed 28 June 2022. https://dtxalliance.org/wp-content/uploads/2021/01/DTA_DTx-Definition-and-Core-Principles.pdf
7. Digital Therapeutics Alliance, 'DTx Product Best Practices'. November (2019). Accessed 29 September 2022. https://dtxalliance.org/wp-content/uploads/2021/01/DTA_DTx-Product-Best-Practices_11.11.19.pdf
8. Latulippe, K., Hamel, C., Giroux, D.: Social health inequalities and eHealth: a literature review with qualitative synthesis of theoretical and empirical studies. J. Med. Internet Res. **19**(4), e6731 (2017). https://doi.org/10.2196/jmir.6731
9. International Electrotechnical Commission.: Medical Devices—Part 2: Guidance on the Application of Usability Engineering to Medical Devices, 1st edn. International Electrotechnical Commission, Geneva, CH (2016). Accessed 14 June 2022. https://www.iso.org/cms/render/live/en/sites/isoorg/contents/data/standard/06/91/69126.html
10. Ravizza, A., Lantada, A., Sánchez, L., Sternini, F., Bignardi, C.: Techniques for usability risk assessment during medical device design. In: Presented at the 12th International Conference on Biomedical Electronics and Devices, June, pp. 207–214 (2022). Accessed 28 June 2022. https://www.scitepress.org/Link.aspx?doi=10.5220/0007483102070214

11. Fox, S., et al.: Co-design of a smartphone app for people living with dementia by applying agile, iterative co-design principles: development and usability study. JMIR MHealth UHealth **10**(1), e24483 (2022). https://doi.org/10.2196/24483
12. Sumner, J., Chong, L.S., Bundele, A., Wei Lim, Y.: Co-designing technology for aging in place: a systematic review. Gerontologist **61**(7), e395–e409 (2021). https://doi.org/10.1093/geront/gnaa064
13. Bjerkan, J., Kane, B., Uhrenfeldt, L., Veie, M., Fossum, M.: Citizen-patient involvement in the development of mHealth technology: protocol for a systematic scoping review. JMIR Res. Protoc. **9**(8), e16781 (2020). https://doi.org/10.2196/16781
14. Godfrey, S.B., Barresi, G.: Video games for positive aging: playfully engaging older adults. In: Scataglini, S., Imbesi, S., Marques, G. (eds.) Internet of Things for Human-Centered Design: Application to Elderly Healthcare, pp. 375–404. Springer Nature, Singapore (2022). https://doi.org/10.1007/978-981-16-8488-3_18
15. Lavallee, D.C., Lee, J.R., Semple, J.L., Lober, W.B., Evans, H.L.: Engaging patients in co-design of mobile health tools for surgical site infection surveillance: implications for research and implementation. Surg. Infect. **20**(7), 535–540 (2019). https://doi.org/10.1089/sur.2019.148
16. Jessen, S., Mirkovic, J., Ruland, C.M.: Creating gameful design in mHealth: a participatory co-design approach. JMIR MHealth UHealth **6**(12), e11579 (2018). https://doi.org/10.2196/11579
17. Ambe, A.H., Brereton, M., Soro, A., Chai, M.Z., Buys, L., Roe, P.: Older people inventing their personal internet of things with the IoT Un-Kit experience. In: Proceedings of the 2019 CHI Conference on Human Factors in Computing Systems, Glasgow Scotland UK, May 2019, pp. 1–15. https://doi.org/10.1145/3290605.3300552
18. Petrushin, A., et al.: IoT-powered monitoring systems for geriatric healthcare: overview. In: Scataglini, S., Imbesi, S., Marques, G. (eds.) Internet of Things for Human-Centered Design: Application to Elderly Healthcare, pp. 99–122. Springer Nature, Singapore (2022). https://doi.org/10.1007/978-981-16-8488-3_6
19. Mesko, B., Győrffy, Z.: The rise of the empowered physician in the digital health era: viewpoint. J. Med. Internet Res. **21**(3), e12490 (2019). https://doi.org/10.2196/12490
20. Zhang, J., Johnson, T.R., Patel, V.L., Paige, D.L., Kubose, T.: Using usability heuristics to evaluate patient safety of medical devices. J. Biomed. Inform. **36**(1), 23–30 (2003). https://doi.org/10.1016/S1532-0464(03)00060-1
21. Stuppia, N., et al.: Risk-based comprehensive usability evaluation of software as a medical device. In: Presented at the 15th International Conference on Health Informatics, June, pp. 454–462 (2022). Accessed 28 June 2022. https://www.scitepress.org/Link.aspx?doi=10.5220/0010825100003123
22. Sternini, F., et al.: Usability assessment of an intraoperative planning software. In: Proceedings of the 14th International Joint Conference on Biomedical Engineering Systems and Technologies, Online Streaming, Select a Country, pp. 483–492 (2021). https://doi.org/10.5220/0010252904830492
23. Donald, M., et al.: A web-based self-management support prototype for adults with chronic kidney disease (My Kidneys My Health): co-design and usability testing. JMIR Form. Res. **5**(2), e22220 (2021). https://doi.org/10.2196/22220
24. Tremblay, M., et al.: Usability of a co-designed ehealth prototype for caregivers: combination study of three frameworks. JMIR Hum. Factors **8**(3), e26532 (2021). https://doi.org/10.2196/26532
25. Khanbhai, M., et al.: Enriching the value of patient experience feedback: web-based dashboard development using co-design and heuristic evaluation. JMIR Hum. Factors **9**(1), e27887 (2022). https://doi.org/10.2196/27887
26. Nielsen, J.: Enhancing the explanatory power of usability heuristics. In: Proceedings of the SIGCHI conference on Human factors in computing systems celebrating interdependence—CHI '94, Boston, Massachusetts, United States, pp. 152–158 (1994). https://doi.org/10.1145/191666.191729

27. International Organization for Standardization.: Medical Devices—Guidance on the Application of ISO 14971, 2nd edn. International Organization for Standardization, Geneva, CH (2020). Accessed 29 June 2022. https://www.iso.org/cms/render/live/en/sites/isoorg/contents/data/standard/07/44/74437.html
28. International Organization for Standardization.: Medical Devices—Information to be Supplied by the Manufacturer, 1st edn. International Organization for Standardization, Geneva, CH (2021). Accessed 29 June 2022. https://www.iso.org/cms/render/live/en/sites/isoorg/contents/data/standard/06/79/67943.html
29. International Electrotechnical Commission.: Medical Devices—Part 1: Application of Usability Engineering to Medical Devices, 1.1. International Electrotechnical Commission, Geneva, CH (2020). Accessed 30 June 2022. https://www.iso.org/cms/render/live/en/sites/isoorg/contents/data/standard/06/31/63179.html
30. International Organization for Standardization.: Medical Devices—Application of Risk Management to Medical Devices, 3rd edn. International Organization for Standardization, Geneva, CH (2019). Accessed 30 June 2022. https://www.iso.org/cms/render/live/en/sites/isoorg/contents/data/standard/07/27/72704.html
31. International Organization for Standardization.: Medical Devices—Quality Management Systems—Requirements for Regulatory Purposes, 3rd edn. International Organization for Standardization, Geneva, CH (2016). Accessed June 30 2022. https://www.iso.org/cms/render/live/en/sites/isoorg/contents/data/standard/05/97/59752.html
32. Pietro, L.D., De Maria, C., Ravizza, A., Ahluwalia, A.: Co-design open-source medical devices: how to minimize the human error using UBORA e-infrastructure. In: Annual International Conference IEEE Engineering in Medicine Biology Society, July, vol. 2019, pp. 3730–3733 (2019). https://doi.org/10.1109/EMBC.2019.8856891

# Phygital Mental Health: Opportunities and Challenges

**Andrea Gaggioli, Antonio Cerasa, and Giacinto Barresi**

## 1 Introduction

Novel interaction technologies can move the boundaries of human experience by generating computer-generated settings. Furthermore, these innovations may intertwine virtuality and reality along a continuum [1, 2] that encompasses different processes and conditions of experiential augmentation: reality can be perceptually enriched by virtual items as in Augmented Reality (AR), and real items can be added to virtuality itself as in Augmented Virtuality (AV). Furthermore, these settings are embraced by the umbrella term of Mixed Reality (MR), even if its (currently debated) definition is shifting: e.g. MR can be considered as a condition where the computer-generated items should behave as physical objects in a real setting when they interact with a user, at least as integrated with the setting.

Among the phenomena belonging to these domains of Extended Reality (XR), where reality and virtuality co-exist through heterogeneous modalities [3], "phygital"

A. Gaggioli (✉)
Research Center in Communication Psychology, Università Cattolica del Sacro Cuore, Milan, Italy
e-mail: andrea.gaggioli@unicatt.it

Applied Technology for Neuro-Psychology Lab, IRCCS Istituto Auxologico Italiano, Milan, Italy

A. Cerasa
Institute for Biomedical Research and Innovation, National Research Council, IRIB-CNR, 98164 Messina, Italy

S. Anna Institute, Crotone, Italy

Pharmacotechnology Documentation and Transfer Unit, Preclinical and Translational Pharmacology, Department of Pharmacy, Health Science and Nutrition, University of Calabria, Arcavacata, Italy

G. Barresi
Rehab Technologies Lab, Istituto Italiano di Tecnologia (IIT), Genova, Italy



S. Scataglini et al. (eds.), *mHealth and Human-Centered Design Towards Enhanced Health, Care, and Well-Being*, Studies in Big Data 120,
https://doi.org/10.1007/978-981-99-3989-3_2

interactions may occur. The attribute of "phygital" is a neologism resulting from the synthesis of two terms—"physical" and "digital"—in various fields like design and marketing [4]. Such a hybrid quality derives from a reality-virtuality convergence enabled by technologies (e.g., the systems for the aforementioned XR, or the pervasive devices for Internet of Things - IoT). These solutions can radically transform any living space (e.g., houses, offices, public spaces, even a city as a whole) by blending real and simulated items or they can enrich a digital setting by establishing continuity with a physical one. As phygital elements, the objects and agents within a technological ecosystem supporting this reality-virtuality fusion can become "programmable interfaces", sources of radically novel experiential classes [5].

Such phygital ecosystems, enacted through common objects and environments enhanced by sensors, displays, and actuators connected to Artificial Intelligence (AI) solutions, can be capable of context awareness, especially through their sensitivity to the presence of individuals and groups. This makes the phygital ecosystem (and, possibly, each component of it) capable of personalizing automated activities or offering natural interaction modalities to their users. Such features make a phygital space a potential ally in mHealth, especially considering the general frameworks of Digital Health. In particular, they can transform the healthcare services alongside the human behaviors through "metanatural" user interfaces, investing the individual with the full capabilities of Connected Care without detaching people from reality.

After a general introduction to phygital interactions, this chapter will focus on potential applications of this paradigm to mental health, paying special attention to the mHealth solutions dedicated to monitor and improve the psychological well-being of people navigating across physical and digital worlds.

## 2 Phygital Convergences and Interactions

The phygital paradigm can be considered as an exemplary result of a general virtual-real convergence trend [6] that can ultimately disclose novel approaches to human-technology interaction in multiple activities of daily living. We can find an ancestor of the most recent developments of this convergence in the Natural User Interfaces—NUIs [7]. Typically, such systems receive commands through the voice or the gestures of their users: this way, a human communicates with a computational system through natural acts that seem to get the user and machine closer. Nevertheless, even if these control modalities seem "natural", their use is not necessarily spontaneous and intuitive in any context [8, 9]. Indeed, gestures based on wide movements of an open hand can be practical in everyday social settings, surely not while the user is a physician carefully moving a laser along a tissue by means of a robotic device for microsurgery [10]. Reality-Based Interaction (RBI) design [11] seems a promising approach to move beyond NUIs. RBI gets inspiration from meaningful actions performed by humans in the real world: they follow concepts of naive physics and they exploit the individual (bodily, social, environmental) awareness and skills that are required for affecting the non-mediated contexts.

Accordingly, RBI systems can be designed to exploit the user's sensorimotor abilities for handling real and virtual objects into a hybrid setting (indeed, AR and MR are considered as one of the RBI concepts), while they provide the user with the expected physical feedback, for instance as visuo-haptic stimulation in surgery [12]. This latter aspect highlights another class of RBI solutions: the Tangible User Interfaces (TUIs) [13], based on physical items with haptic functions for collecting the input and, possibly, releasing the output of processes underlying Human–Machine Interactions (HMIs) or the sub-class of Human–Computer Interactions (HCIs). Historically, we can say that these solutions constitute a premise for the effort of establishing a bridge between different dimensions of reality and virtuality. Such a bridge relies on affordances sustaining the overlap of physical and digital items interacting with a human being. On the other hand, the behavior of these hybrid objects depends on multimodal data collected from the setting and from the user: interestingly, it is possible to exploit their virtual component to enable an intuitive control of their physical features. An example (in surgery, again) of this potential is offered by a Brain-Computer Interface (BCI) used to monitor the attention of a physician for representing the possibility to activate a laser through a "retractable" AR scalpel providing visuo-haptic feedback [14]. Thus, such a brain-sensitive digital device held as a physical tool is another demonstration of the versatility of the innovations derived from the virtuality-reality convergence trend, "infusing" a Human–Robot Interaction (HRI) system with neurocognitive data represented through AR items to facilitate a physical activity.

Overall, embodying the representation of multimodal data through TUIs constitutes a premise for further developments as the aforementioned phygital interaction. Phygital spaces work as hybrid settings where it is possible to physically interact with virtual items, and virtually with physical ones [5]. The latter category enlists computational devices embodied and embedded in living environments (from furniture to wearable gadgets), which become informational ecosystems characterized by a continuous and bidirectional exchange of data between the real and the digital world, de facto transforming our own experience [15]. Through innovation in technological infrastructures, especially after the pandemic outbreak [16], human-technology confluence paradigms like phygital interaction literally exploded for providing solutions to get people closer within the same hybrid settings to perform shared activities. This happened, for instance, in contexts like work and education [17, 18]. However, phygital systems certainly emerged in heterogeneous applications before the COVID-19. For instance, Nakazawa and Tokuda [19] proposed a setup where a mouse can be moved across a paper-made geographic map for selecting the information visualized on digital devices (like showing touristic locations on a smartphone according to the position of the mouse on the map). The authors consider it a phygital interface as a special kind of TUI where physical objects can control and map the digital objects (with a clear separation between the place where digital information is displayed).

More recent peculiar concepts have been proposed as the "phygital play" in [20]: a mixed reality-based projected playground where people and robots can physically interact. This approach can also facilitate the design and development of games involving both digital and physical items in a shared setting, as in mixed reality-based robotic games (MRRGs) [21]. In general, the term "phygital" defines a space where physical and digital items can converge to inspire innovations in interconnectivity patterns across reality and virtuality. This definition approaches one of the metaverse as a digital world with physical connections [22].

Overall, the potential of phygital systems is indubitably versatile, as demonstrated in different domains, from tourism to industry to healthcare [23–25]. In the latter case, such an approach can be especially useful for managing chronic conditions and predicting their progress or the therapeutic outcome through (environmental and wearable) sensor networks and intelligent systems, enabling user-centered paradigms of ubiquitous interaction and mobile computing [26, 27]. These approaches perfectly work within the field of digital health services [28], especially considering the opportunity of pervasively engaging the patients for motivating health-related activities and clinical compliance. Examples of this application of phygital features have occurred already in the past decade, as in [29] about the Active Parks project, promoting physical exercise habits of older and sedentary people in urban spaces through co-designed playful phygital artefacts and games (even bridging the generation gap, a crucial drive in motivating elder people) [30].

Interestingly, the exploitation of phygital solutions for engaging people can take precious suggestions from a field where this approach is frequently explored for involving the customers: the marketing [31]. Indeed, the difficulties in academic conceptualization of the phygital label are sometimes faced by marketing channel strategies exploiting physical-digital solutions. However, this domain offers an intensive dialectics that can drive the organization of the potential of phygital interactions within a holistic framework to manage the customer experience. An interesting example (Fig. 1) of this approach is the Social Swipe [32]. The Social Swipe is based on a credit card swipe machine inserted into an interactive public screen. People can read messages on the screen, inviting the observers to "Feed Them" or "Free Them" (referring to people in difficult conditions). After approaching the screen, the individual attracted by such messages can swipe their credit card as a blade for cutting a slide of bread or the ropes tying two hands. Through this, a donation of 2 euros is made for (respectively) providing people with food or for returning children to their life. Such an engaging concept of interaction exploits a connection between an intuitive physical gestures for manipulating a digital resource, as in phygital paradigms.

This type of effort to shape customer experience can occur in case of user experience and patient experience as well, envisioning how to capture the individual attention by proposing compelling smart responses from interactive and connected objects.

Considering practical aspects, phygital systems offer intriguing options for engaging people in digital health and mobile health (mHealth) contexts. Within this framework, mobile systems can work to collect information that can be exploited for identifying the current state of the person within the phygital setting, possibly generating information for adaptive and personalized interactions with the surroundings—an extremely useful feature for frail people with increasing needs, as in case of elderly [27]. Furthermore, they can become sources of potential digital and phygital biomarkers [33, 34] that can work as indices of the current and future conditions

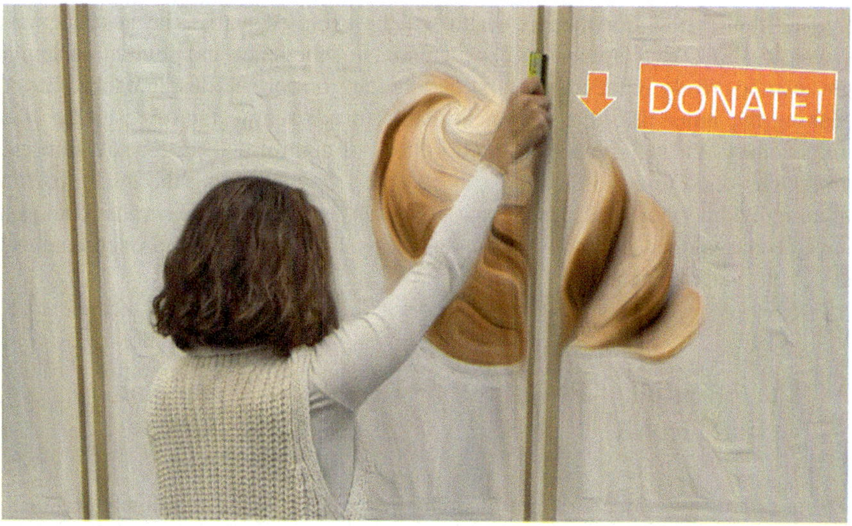


**Fig. 1** An example of a potentially phygital screen, representing the concept of the Misereor Social Swipe. https://www.youtube.com/watch?v=zVuWtWZh4oQ

of a person. Indeed, during the human interactions with phygital items and spaces, it is possible to make the user choices and actions the information for reaching a diagnosis or a prognosis, or even planning a change in the furniture of the home for easing the activities of daily living (ADLs) of a specific person. The advantages of making "person-aware" environments can be further enriched by the concept of "reality as an app": a scenario where each item can be potentially "programmed" through physical and digital actions to enable new forms of experiences.

On the other hand, we should consider how future (and futuristic) evolutions of this scenario could make it difficult to distinguish the digital and physical aspects of experience while we move back and forth between these two dimensions, possibly intertwining different levels of virtuality and reality in daily living contexts. Indeed, any continuity across these worlds may generate a holistic flow of experience for the users. In particular, wearable and environmental sensors can augment the human capability to be informed by the surroundings and to alter them through solutions for visualization and actuation that extend the individual understanding, will, and mood (thus, involuntarily) to the physical reality in terms of shapes, colors, sounds, and any potential feedback released by a device. However, we cannot depict such a complex situation as a chaotic mesh of simulated and real items, a context where virtuality projects the inner thoughts and feelings of any person in the real setting. This potential future complexity is just an expression of the same premise for exploiting the current and upcoming solutions merging physical and digital worlds according to a goal-oriented human-centered design [35, 36].

The implications for mental health will be explored across the next sections, discussing how the relationships between human experience and phygital technologies can positively influence the first by a research-informed design of the second. Making the inner life of a person available to a machine for representing it or influencing it through physical-digital options of control and feedback constitutes a precious opportunity. Indeed, it can be a way for improving the quality of life of an individual that needs to manage their own well-being in ways that could not have been imagined before the "phygital magics" ignited the mind of researchers, designers, and clinicians.

## 3 The Potential of Phygital Experiences for Enhancing Mental Health

The use of advanced technologies and mobile tools in the prevention and treatment of psychological conditions is an increasing trend. However, most research in cyber-psychology/cyber-therapy so far has focused on specific technology [37], such as VR/AR, mobile tools, and biosensors, while the development of scenarios in which these different tools and services are *integrated* into a "phygital mHealth ecosystem" is still lacking.

To advance this vision, however, considering the patient's experience journey (and of relevant stakeholders, i.e., mental health professionals, healthcare service providers, etc.) is critical to ensure the successful implementation of a phygital strategy in mental health. For example, the development of a mobile system that uses biosensors and artificial intelligence should carefully consider eventual limitations in understanding and using technology, etc. The phygital health experience should align with the needs and expectations of final users. In this context, the overarching objective should not be innovating for innovation's sake, but to understand the need for changing existing practices, i.e., by identifying the specific advantages (and drawbacks) of creating a system/service that blends a physical and digital health experience together. As phygital scenarios in mental health are still embryonic, in what follows we will analyze how the cyber-physical system could be applied in each phase/level of care.

From this perspective, some examples of phygital solutions for mental health can be inspired from the field of marketing, where this technological paradigm is advancing fast, and more specifically, from the emerging literature on phygital customer experience. But how legitimate it is to bring these two apparently distant domains closer together? To answer this question, it should be noted that although the focus on patient's experience is a recent concern, it is a significant one, being recognized as one of the three key dimensions of quality in healthcare, alongside clinical effectiveness, and patient safety [38]. Furthermore, patient experience is positively correlated to health outcomes, healthcare resource use, and medication and treatment adherence [39]. As noted by McCarthy and Coll. [39], patient experience should be a principal goal along with delivering performance improvement and meeting constraints, as an efficient and compliant process does not necessarily mean a good experience will be delivered.

Therefore, in the same way, that phygital applications in marketing are expected to play a crucial role in enhancing customer's experience, so their "translation" in the field of healthcare could inspire new strategies for enhancing patient's experience. It should also be noticed that such fruitful "contamination" between marketing and healthcare fields is not new: for example, the concept of patient engagement is borrowed from the marketing conceptualization of consumer engagement. This posits that making patients/clients co-producers of their health can enhance their satisfaction with the healthcare system as well as their responsibility in both care and prevention [40].

## *3.1 Mental Health Promotion and Illness Prevention*

The World Health Organization defines mental health as "a state of well-being in which every individual realizes his or her own potential, can cope with the normal stresses of life, can work productively and fruitfully, and is able to make a contribution to her or his community" [40]. In this, the absence of mental disorder does not necessarily mean the presence of good mental health [41]. Specifically, according to WHO, while prevention is concerned with avoiding disease, mental health promotion aims at fostering individual competencies, resources, and psychological strengths, and to strengthen community assets to prevent mental disorder and enhance well-being and quality of life for people and communities [41]. In this context, building positive health behaviors and maintaining psychological well-being are essential for promoting mental health and illness prevention. For example, it is well-known that lifestyle factors play a significant role in determining both physical and mental health [42]. These include, for example, nutrition, physical activity, sleep, alcohol and smoking and social support/interaction. In this sense, the emergence of phygital health could be used to positively influence lifestyle factors to prevent or improve physical and mental health, with particular emphasis on food, diet, sleep and exercise. This can be considered as an evolution of digital mental health approaches through the merging of (interconnected) computer-generated and physical items [43, 44].

In particular, phygital experiences can improve the well-being and social connectedness, as demonstrated by mental health apps helping people to engage in potentially uneasy discussions on their wellness, facilitating the interaction with care professionals [45].

### 3.2 *Early Detection and Diagnostics*

In the area of secondary prevention, early detection and intervention are key to reduce chronicity, mortality, disability and the socio-economic burden associated with mental disorders. Phygital ecosystems may offer novel, integrated and personalized strategies to provide timelier and more accurate diagnostics.

For example, wearable sensors allow us to measure human physiologic parameters in a continuous, real-time, and nonintrusive manner. These data can be combined with information gathered from other Internet of Things devices disseminated in homes, public spaces, vehicles, and healthcare facilities. Thanks to the increasing pervasiveness of these tools, it is possible to collect a wide range of physio-behavioral information, which can be used to measure i.e. physical activity and coordination, cognitive efficiency, emotions, level of social interaction, mood states and stress levels [46].

Furthermore, thanks to the increasingly widespread adoption of electronic health records, it is possible to apply AI-based prediction algorithms for the automatic detection of critical mental health events for example, suicide, self-harm and first episode psychosis [47].

Conversational agents (Fig. 2) can further extend the range of phygital tools that can be used to gather diagnostic information [47]. For example, conversational AIs have interviewed patients about symptoms for PTSD with a high level of patient acceptance. Conversational AI has been piloted across numerous clinically relevant groups such as clinical depression [48] and adolescent stress [49]. Other researchers are also exploring the potential of using conversational AI in combination with virtual reality and affective computing to extend the "empathetic abilities" of the virtual therapeutic assistant. One of the most advanced examples of this approach is SimSensei kiosk, a "virtual health agent" designed to create an engaging face-to-face interaction where the user feels comfortable talking and sharing information [50]. According to the authors, the virtual character can autonomously engage in an interview with a human subject by sensing and interpreting nonverbal signals (i.e., facial expressions, gestures, and vocal prosody) to make determinations about the person's level of anxiety. Obviously, tangible (especially robotic) conversational agents like coaches for the elderly can be even more impactful on the individual engagement and well-being, demonstrating the full capabilities of the phygital interaction paradigms [51, 52].

### 3.3 *Accessibility and Inclusion*

Certainly, phygital systems demonstrated their capability to engage people besides neuromotor impairments, possibly facilitating rehabilitative processes. Indeed, through haptic control of physical and digital items, it is possible for a person with a Neuro-Developmental Disorder (NDD) to interact with a game such as Reflex [53], a

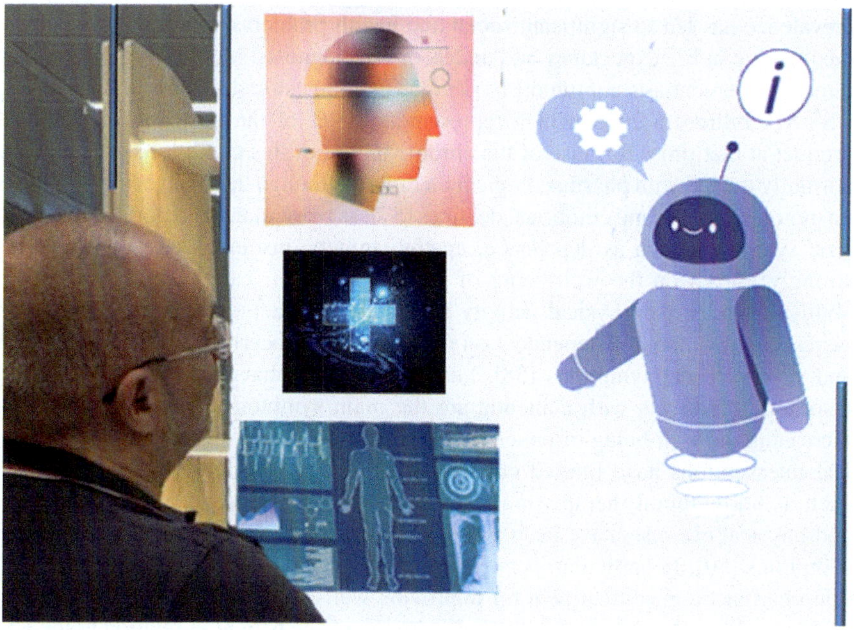

**Fig. 2** An example of a potential conversational agent for diagnostics

mobile training application integrating a mirrored camera. Through a cross-platform app for smartphones and tablets, Reflex exploits tracking solutions for connecting physical and digital items, enabling novel opportunities for learning and training in the case of NDD, showing high potential in terms of accessibility and inclusion. This can work as a premise for developing intuitive solutions for rehabilitation and therapy dedicated to people with neurocognitive impairments (as a preliminary step for any behavioral treatment). Interestingly, the aspect of inclusion is emphasized in other studies [54] based on environments enabling collaborative phygital activities for children with and without disabilities through actions that can be performed regardless of cognitive impairments [55].

Beyond the valuable impact of accessibility and inclusion on mental health, phygital solutions facilitate the fruition of tools for mental healthcare and, in particular, cognitive stimulation and rehabilitation. The next sub-section will present a potential scenario of applications in this direction.

### 3.4 A Potential Scenario: From Virtual to Phygital Applications in Dementia

Nowadays, there are over 55 million people worldwide living with dementia, which will continue to increase, estimated to reach 139 million in 2050 [56]. This high prevalence has led to significant social and health problems which will rise due to the increase in life expectancy and under- or misdiagnosis. Moreover, the economic impact of dementia is continuously rising. The total estimated worldwide cost was US$ 818 billion in 2015, which represented 1.09% of the global gross domestic product at that time. Because of the chronic nature of this condition, patients were normally treated with pharmacological therapies, although these have limited effects on motor, cognitive and emotional declines [57]. In particular, behavioral and psychiatric symptoms such as depression, apathy, anxiety, insomnia, and hallucination, strongly impact on the well-being of patients and their caregivers, limiting their ability to undertake physical activity and social interactions. Basically, they felt being disconnected and dependent on others, which exacerbates negative emotions and psychological symptoms [58]. For this reason, behavioral and psychological disorders in patients with dementia are the main symptoms to be considered for increasing the well-being of patients and their caregivers. Until now, pharmacological interventions have limited effects, whilst non-pharmacological interventions, such as horticultural therapy, music therapy, animal-assisted therapy, art therapy, and physical exercise, have been demonstrated effective in reducing psychological symptoms [59]. In particular, person-centered care has been recognized as the best non-pharmacological treatment for improving well-being in patients with dementia [60], given that this recognizes the individuality of the patient in relation to the attitudes and practices that surround them [61]. Patients with dementia feel better when engaged in meaningful activities, such as social participation, and work-related activities, which improve the individual's sense of autonomy and identity. The person-centered care approach recognizes the unmet needs of patients that are the basis of behavioral disorders. When psychological needs were satisfied, behavioral symptoms tend to decrease [62], and such reductions have been effective in reducing the need for neuroleptics [63]. Recent meta-analytic studies [60] showed that intensive person-centered care treatments significantly improved neuropsychiatric symptoms and quality of life when compared with usual care in people with dementia. Up to now, the application of existing non-pharmacological interventions to patients with dementia is difficult. To overcome these issues, multisensory VR platforms have been proposed to improve cognitive function and behavioral symptoms in patients with dementia. Serious Games are considered motivating by patients with mild cognitive impairment (MCI) and Alzheimer's disease (AD), stimulating a number of cognitive functions, such as attention and memory and visuo-spatial abilities [64]. The motivation to use VR in dementia is related to the possibility to customize the virtual scenarios and the activities, to make them more engaging. Individuals with dementia are more engaged by activities and stimuli that match their interests and personal history [65]. The main target is to create solutions for increasing the feeling of "engagement" that has been shown to have positive effects on functional abilities and quality of life in patients with dementia [66]. The psychological needs of individuals with dementia include five factors: comfort, identity, attachment, occupation, and inclusion [67]. For this reason, to be effective, VR-related tools should be customized to the personal needs of people with dementia. In this regard, Kim et al.

[68] developed a fully immersive audiovisual experience of different virtual environments. Music, sound, movies and photos were added, in addition to anecdotes and verbal cues. To meet the psychological needs of older people, the content consisted of different environments for fostering positive emotions. The VR content was developed to fulfill every psychological need of patients with dementia. Indeed, patients were engaged in a virtual environment where they had to give train tickets to station attendants, drink black herbal tea, receive family gifts or photos, and watch naturalistic and familiar scenes. Manera et al. [69] developed an image-based rendered environment to train selective and sustained attention in VR settings. They found that individuals with mild cognitive disorders or AD had lower level of anxiety, discomfort, and fatigue and higher levels of satisfaction with image-based VR exercises compared to standard exercises. Finally, McEwen et al. [63] evaluated the feasibility and safety of an exercise-based VR training program characterized by a serious game in a single patient with dementia. In agreement with previous studies, they found that VR exercise is an enjoyable, safe, and feasible intervention for this kind of patient. Despite these promising results, the usability of the VR systems developed for patients with dementia are characterized by several limitations. (1) The experience length. Most of the studies established a variable duration from 5 to 15 min. This time is strongly dependent on patients' feelings since they typically experience decreased comfort with technological devices. (2) The weight of the head-mounted displays. (3) The interaction between body motion and visual stimuli. Indeed, individuals displayed difficulties operating the VR with hand movements mostly likely because of motor and cognitive deficits of the older patients. (4) Reduced sensory acuity. The VR environment requires active movements merging together auditory and visual senses. This is obviously limited in this kind of patients who typically experience reduced attention and visuo-spatial deficits. (5) Dizziness or nausea during the VR immersion, is often reported in older individuals. Thus it is mandatory to develop different solutions for stimulating cognitive and emotional engagement in people with dementia, extending beyond the standard VR-related setting to a new phygital concept of spaces.

The exploitation of phygital solutions for improving behavioral symptoms in patients with dementia is still lacking yet. As recently stated by Matsangidou et al. [70] the main attributes of a virtual (or phygital) environment for patients with dementia should have: (1) a simple interactions modality; (2) visible visual targets and continuous feedback; (3) personalized virtual environments; (4) personalized range of movements. With this in mind, there is a need to extract from this emerging phygital technology, every solution that may satisfy the specific psychological needs of patients in the context of real usability of VR-related tools making environments "person/caregiver-aware". The next phygital applications for mental health in dementia should define new strategies for enhancing the patient's experience by means of:

(a) conversational agents able to extend the "empathetic abilities" of the real (or virtual) therapists;

(b) AI-based prediction algorithms integrated into the phygital environment for the automatic detection of critical behavioral events (hallucination, apathy etc.);
(c) a new generation of visual systems for AR (instead of the most famous VR goggles) enriching the environment even with the presence of another person.

## 4 Conclusion

This chapter introduced the perspective of a convergence of physical and digital worlds within the framework of phygital interaction. Such a perspective is demonstrated to be quite fertile in offering novel ways for easing human activities and improving the quality of life for people with health issues. In particular, this chapter discussed the opportunities in mental health domains—from assessment to treatment—with a special focus on the elderly within a scenario including conversational agents that can enrich the daily life of a person through their own phygital quality, as a bridge between digital and physical services adjusted according to the individual commands and conditions. Indeed, this approach demonstrates the possibility of providing people with a "programmable" environment where mHealth solutions play a fundamental role as portable interfaces that integrate the possibility of interaction offered by socially and haptically reactive items. Further research will be required for devising and validating phygital solutions for mental health, considering how the technologies encompassed by this interaction paradigm can be designed for making our setting more "human".

## References

1. Milgram, P., Kishino, F.: A taxonomy of mixed reality visual displays. IEICE Trans. Inf. Syst. **77**(12), 1321–1329 (1994)
2. Skarbez, R., Smith, M., Whitton, M.C.: Revisiting milgram and Kishino's reality-virtuality continuum. Front. Virtual Real. **2**, 27 (2021)
3. Chuah, S.H-W.: Why and who will adopt extended reality technology? Literature review, synthesis, and future research agenda. Literature Review. Synthesis, and Future Research Agenda, 13 December (2018)
4. Soloviov, E., Danilov, A.: The beginning of phygital world. South Asian J. Eng. Technol. **10** (2020)
5. Gaggioli, A.: Phygital spaces: when atoms meet bits. Cyberpsychol. Behav. Soc. Netw. **20**(12), 774–774 (2017)
6. Lehman-Wilzig, S.N.: Virtuality and reality: two sides of the same coin. In: Virtuality and Humanity, pp 243–260. Springer (2021)
7. Liu, W.: Natural user interface-next mainstream product user interface. In: 2010 IEEE 11th International Conference on Computer-Aided Industrial Design & Conceptual Design 1. IEEE, pp. 203–205 (2010)
8. Malizia, A., Bellucci, A.: The artificiality of natural user interfaces. Commun. ACM **55**(3), 36–38 (2012)
9. Norman, D.A.: Natural user interfaces are not natural. Interactions **17**(3), 6–10 (2010)

10. Barresi, G., Deshpande, N., Mattos, L.S., Brogni, A., Guastini, L., Peretti, G., Caldwell, D.G.: Comparative usability and performance evaluation of surgeon interfaces in laser phonomicrosurgery. In: 2013 IEEE/RSJ International Conference on Intelligent Robots and Systems. IEEE, pp. 3610–3615 (2013)
11. Jacob, R.J., Girouard, A., Hirshfield, L.M., Horn, M.S., Shaer, O., Solovey, E.T., Zigelbaum, J.: Reality-based interaction: a framework for post-WIMP interfaces. In: Proceedings of the SIGCHI Conference on Human Factors in Computing Systems, pp. 201–210 (2008)
12. Olivieri, E., Barresi, G., Caldwell, D.G., Mattos, L.S.: Haptic feedback for control and active constraints in contactless laser surgery: concept, implementation, and evaluation. IEEE Trans. Haptics **11**(2), 241–254 (2017)
13. Holmquist, L.E., Zuckerman, O., Ballagas, R., Ishii, H., Ryokai, K., Zhang, H.: The future of tangible user interfaces. In: Extended Abstracts of the 2019 CHI Conference on Human Factors in Computing Systems, pp. 1–6 (2019)
14. Barresi, G., Olivieri, E., Caldwell, D.G., Mattos, L.S.: Brain-controlled AR feedback design for user's training in surgical HRI. In: 2015 IEEE International Conference on Systems, Man, and Cybernetics. IEEE, pp 1116–1121 (2015)
15. Riva, G., Baños, R.M., Botella, C., Mantovani, F., Gaggioli, A.: Transforming experience: the potential of augmented reality and virtual reality for enhancing personal and clinical change. Front. Psych. **7**, 164 (2016)
16. Allam, Z., Jones, D.S.: Future (post-COVID) digital, smart and sustainable cities in the wake of 6G: digital twins, immersive realities and new urban economies. Land Use Policy **101**, 105201 (2021)
17. Burova, N.V., Molodkova, E.B., Nikolaenko, A.V., Popazova, O.A.: Remote work as a societal incentive for creativity: phygital initiative for self-actualization. In: International Conference on Professional Culture of the Specialist of the Future, pp. 168–181. Springer (2021)
18. Chaturvedi, S., Purohit, S., Verma, M.: Effective teaching practices for success during COVID 19 pandemic: towards phygital learning. Front. Educ. **6**, 646557 (2021). https://doi.org/10.3389/feduc.2021.646557
19. Nakazawa, J., Tokuda, H.: Phygital map: Accessing digital multimedia from physical map. In: 21st International Conference on Advanced Information Networking and Applications Workshops (AINAW'07). IEEE, pp. 368–373 (2007)
20. Lupetti, M.L., Piumatti, G., Rossetto, F.: Phygital play HRI in a new gaming scenario. In: 2015 7th International Conference on Intelligent Technologies for Interactive Entertainment (INTETAIN). IEEE, pp. 17–21 (2015)
21. Prattico, F.G., Lamberti, F.: Mixed-reality robotic games: design guidelines for effective entertainment with consumer robots. IEEE Consum. Electron. Mag. **10**(1), 6–16 (2020)
22. Yoon, K., Kim, S.-K., Jeong, S.P., Choi, J.-H.: Interfacing cyber and physical worlds: introduction to IEEE 2888 standards. In: 2021 IEEE International Conference on Intelligent Reality (ICIR). IEEE, pp. 49–50 (2021)
23. Czwick, C., Anderl, R.: Cyber-physical twins-definition, conception and benefit. Procedia CIRP **90**, 584–588 (2020)
24. Stankov, U., Gretzel, U.: Tourism 4.0 technologies and tourist experiences: a human-centered design perspective. Inf. Technol. Tour. **22**(3), 477–488 (2020)
25. Gregory, D.: Healthcare Goes Digital: Designing for the Convergence of the Digital and Physical Environment—Implications for Design Professionals. SAGE Publications Sage CA, Los Angeles, CA (2022)
26. Voigt, I., Inojosa, H., Dillenseger, A., Haase, R., Akgün, K., Ziemssen, T.: Digital twins for multiple sclerosis. Front. Immunol. **12**, 1556 (2021)
27. Barresi, G., Zenzeri, J., Tessadori, J., Laffranchi, M., Semprini, M., Michieli, L.D.: Neurogerontechnologies: applications and opportunities. In: Internet of Things for Human-Centered Design, pp. 123–153. Springer (2022)
28. Andreoni, G., Caiani, E.G., Castaldini, N.: Digital health services through patient empowerment: classification, current state and preliminary impact assessment by health Pod systems. Appl. Sci. **12**(1), 359 (2021)

29. Tsekleves, E., Gradinar, A., Darby, A., Smith, M.: Active parks:'Phygital' urban games for sedentary and older people. In: Games for Health, pp 140–143. Springer (2014)
30. Godfrey, S.B., Barresi, G.: Video games for positive aging: playfully engaging older adults. In: Internet of Things for Human-Centered Design, pp. 375–404. Springer (2022)
31. Batat, W.: What does phygital really mean? A conceptual introduction to the phygital customer experience (PH-CX) framework. J. Strateg. Market. 1–24 (2022)
32. Huarng, K.-H., Bresciani, S., Ferraris, A.: Experiential interaction design model. J. Bus. Res. **118**, 486–490 (2020)
33. Wright, J.M., Regele, O.B., Kourtis, L.C., Pszenny, S.M., Sirkar, R., Kovalchick, C., Jones, G.B.: Evolution of the digital biomarker ecosystem. Dig. Med. **3**(4), 154 (2017)
34. Barresi, G., Pacchierotti, C., Laffranchi, M., De Michieli, L.: Beyond digital twins: phygital twins for neuroergonomics in human-robot interaction. Front. Neurorobot. 138 (2022)
35. Carella, G., Arquilla, V., Zurlo, F., Tamburello, M.: Phygital experiences design (2019)
36. Mele, C., Russo-Spena, T., Tregua, M., Amitrano, C.C.: The millennial customer journey: a Phygital mapping of emotional, behavioural, and social experiences. J. Consum. Market. (2021)
37. Andrews, C., Southworth, M.K., Silva, J.N., Silva, J.R.: Extended reality in medical practice. Curr. Treat. Options Cardiovasc. Med. **21**(4), 1–12 (2019)
38. Coulter, A., Fitzpatrick, R., Cornwell, J.: Measures of patients' experience in hospital: purpose, methods and uses. Citeseer (2009)
39. McCarthy, S., O'Raghallaigh, P., Woodworth, S., Lim, Y.L., Kenny, L.C., Adam, F.: An integrated patient journey mapping tool for embedding quality in healthcare service reform. J. Decis. Syst. **25**(sup1), 354–368 (2016)
40. Bosio, A.C.: Patient engagement: the key to redesign the exchange between the demand and supply for healthcare in the era of active ageing. In: Active Ageing and Healthy Living: A Human Centered Approach in Research and Innovation as Source of Quality of Life , vol. 203, p. 85 (2014)
41. Herrman, H., Saxena, S., Moodie, R.: Promoting Mental Health: Concepts, Emerging Evidence, Practice: A Report of the World Health Organization, Department of Mental Health and Substance Abuse in collaboration with the Victorian Health Promotion Foundation and the University of Melbourne. World Health Organization (2005)
42. Walsh, R.: Lifestyle and mental health. Am. Psychol. **66**(7), 579 (2011)
43. Rudd, B.N., Beidas, R.S.: Digital mental health: the answer to the global mental health crisis? JMIR Mental Health **7**(6), e18472 (2020)
44. Drissi, N., Ouhbi, S., Serhani, M.A., Marques, G., de la Torre Díez, I.: Connected mental health solutions: global attitudes, preferences, and concerns. Telemed. e-Health (2022)
45. Veer, E., Dobele, A.: Big boys don't cry [Offline]: the phygital disconnect between online and offline mental wellness engagement. J. Strateg. Market. 1–21 (2021)
46. Monteith, S., Glenn, T., Geddes, J., Severus, E., Whybrow, P.C., Bauer, M.: Internet of things issues related to psychiatry. Int. J. Bipolar Disorders **9**(1), 1–9 (2021)
47. Miner, A.S., Shah, N., Bullock, K.D., Arnow, B.A., Bailenson, J., Hancock, J.: Key considerations for incorporating conversational AI in psychotherapy. Front. Psych. **10**, 746 (2019)
48. Fitzpatrick, K.K., Darcy, A., Vierhile, M.: Delivering cognitive behavior therapy to young adults with symptoms of depression and anxiety using a fully automated conversational agent (Woebot): a randomized controlled trial. JMIR Mental Health **4**(2), e7785 (2017)
49. Huang, J., Li, Q., Xue, Y., Cheng, T., Xu, S., Jia, J., Feng, L.: Teenchat: a chatterbot system for sensing and releasing adolescents' stress. In: International Conference on Health Information Science, pp. 133–145. Springer (2015)
50. Völkel, S.T., Schoedel, R., Kaya, L., Mayer, S.: User perceptions of extraversion in chatbots after repeated use. In: CHI Conference on Human Factors in Computing Systems, pp. 1–18 (2022)
51. Russo, A., D'Onofrio, G., Gangemi, A., Giuliani, F., Mongiovi, M., Ricciardi, F., Greco, F., Cavallo, F., Dario, P., Sancarlo, D.: Dialogue systems and conversational agents for patients with dementia: The human–robot interaction. Rejuvenation Res. **22**(2), 109–120 (2019)

52. El Kamali, M., Angelini, L., Caon, M., Andreoni, G., Khaled, O.A., Mugellini, E.: Towards the NESTORE e-Coach: a tangible and embodied conversational agent for older adults. In: Proceedings of the 2018 ACM International Joint Conference and 2018 International Symposium on Pervasive and Ubiquitous Computing and Wearable Computers, pp. 1656–1663 (2018)
53. Spitale, M., Gelsomini, M., Beccaluva, E., Viola, L., Garzotto, F.: Meeting the needs of people with neuro-developmental disorder through a phygital approach. In: Proceedings of the 13th Biannual Conference of the Italian SIGCHI Chapter: Designing the next interaction, pp. 1–10 (2019)
54. Spitale, M., Piselli, A., Garzotto, F., Del Curto, B.: Designing phygital activities in a smart multisensorial room: a collaborative cognitive environment for children with and without disabilities. In: DeSForM 2019. Beyond Intelligence, pp. 140–148 (2019)
55. Gelsomini, M., Spitale, M., Garzotto, F.: Phygital interfaces for people with intellectual disability: an exploratory study at a social care center. Multim. Tools Appl. **80**(26), 34843–34874 (2021)
56. Nichols, E., Steinmetz, J.D., Vollset, S.E., Fukutaki, K., Chalek, J., Abd-Allah, F., Abdoli, A., Abualhasan, A., Abu-Gharbieh, E., Akram, T.T.: Estimation of the global prevalence of dementia in 2019 and forecasted prevalence in 2050: an analysis for the global burden of disease study 2019. Lancet Public Health **7**(2), e105–e125 (2022)
57. Bessey, L.J., Walaszek, A.: Management of behavioral and psychological symptoms of dementia. Curr. Psychiatry Rep. **21**(8), 1–11 (2019)
58. Tible, O.P., Riese, F., Savaskan, E., von Gunten, A.: Best practice in the management of behavioural and psychological symptoms of dementia. Ther. Adv. Neurol. Disord. **10**(8), 297–309 (2017)
59. Weiss, J.C.: A life worth living: practical strategies for reducing depression in older adults. Am. J. Art Ther. **38**(4), 118 (2000)
60. Kim, S.K., Park, M.: Effectiveness of person-centered care on people with dementia: a systematic review and meta-analysis. Clin. Interv. Aging **12**, 381 (2017)
61. Kitwood, T., Bredin, K.: Towards a theory of dementia care: personhood and well-being. Ageing Soc. **12**(3), 269–287 (1992)
62. Sloane, P.D., Hoeffer, B., Mitchell, C.M., McKenzie, D.A., Barrick, A.L., Rader, J., Stewart, B.J., Talerico, K.A., Rasin, J.H., Zink, R.C.: Effect of person-centered showering and the towel bath on bathing-associated aggression, agitation, and discomfort in nursing home residents with dementia: a randomized, controlled trial. J. Am. Geriatr. Soc. **52**(11), 1795–1804 (2004)
63. McEwen, D., Taillon-Hobson, A., Bilodeau, M., Sveistrup, H., Finestone, H.: Two-week virtual reality training for dementia: Single-case feasibility study. J. Rehabil. Res. Dev. **51**(7), 1069 (2014)
64. McCallum, S., Boletsis, C.: Dementia games: a literature review of dementia-related serious games. In: International Conference on Serious Games Development and Applications, pp. 15–27. Springer (2013)
65. Cohen-Mansfield, J., Thein, K., Dakheel-Ali, M., Marx, M.S.: The underlying meaning of stimuli: impact on engagement of persons with dementia. Psychiatry Res. **177**(1–2), 216–222 (2010)
66. González-Salvador, T., Lyketsos, C.G., Baker, A., Hovanec, L., Roques, C., Brandt, J., Steele, C.: Quality of life in dementia patients in long-term care. Int. J. Geriatr. Psychiatry **15**(2), 181–189 (2000)
67. Kitwood, T.M., Kitwood. T.: Dementia Reconsidered: The Person Comes First, vol. 20. Open University Press Buckingham (1997)
68. Kim, J.-H., Park, S., Lim, H.: Developing a virtual reality for people with dementia in nursing homes based on their psychological needs: a feasibility study. BMC Geriatr. **21**(1), 1–10 (2021)
69. Manera, V., Chapoulie, E., Bourgeois, J., Guerchouche, R., David, R., Ondrej, J., Drettakis, G., Robert, P.: A feasibility study with image-based rendered virtual reality in patients with mild cognitive impairment and dementia. PLoS ONE **11**(3), e0151487 (2016)
70. Matsangidou, M., Frangoudes, F., Schiza, E., Neokleous, K.C., Papayianni, E., Xenari, K., Avraamides, M., Pattichis, C.S. Participatory design and evaluation of virtual reality physical rehabilitation for people living with dementia. Virtual Real. 1–18 (2022)

# Data Uncertainty and m-Health Interaction Design for Aging People

**Alessandro Pollini, Sara Casaccia, Nicole Morresi, and Lorenzo Scalise**

## 1 Introduction

Designing interactions for elderly people is the focus of multidisciplinary research initiatives integrating the applied psychology, design research, and IT engineering perspectives, addressing both the development of an evidence-based interaction and coaching conceptual framework and the methodology for data validation and interpretation [1–3]. In particular the aging psychology has widely addressed the investigation of the changes that aging makes to the human factors [4–7], also with relation to the exploration of novel interaction paradigms and the adoption of multiple devices [8]. Interactive technologies may foster the benefits to maintain physically active, socially, and mentally stimulated [9] in aging people since they may convey digital services enabling functional, relational, and meaningful personal experiences.

More importantly, interacting products and digital services, which are pervasively part of everyday life [10], when designated for the elderly require to be wisely designed according to real-world people experience, their needs, expectations, abilities, and limitations [10, 11].

A. Pollini (✉)
BSD Design, Via Lazzaretto 19, 20156 Milan, Italy
e-mail: alessandro.pollini@bsdesign.eu

S. Casaccia · N. Morresi · L. Scalise
Dipartimento di Ingegneria Industriale e Scienze Matematiche (DIISM), Università Politecnica Delle Marche, Via Brecce Bianche, 60131 Ancona, Italy
e-mail: s.casaccia@staff.univpm.it

N. Morresi
e-mail: n.morresi@pm.univpm.it

L. Scalise
e-mail: l.scalise@staff.univpm.it

 
S. Scataglini et al. (eds.), *mHealth and Human-Centered Design Towards Enhanced Health, Care, and Well-Being*, Studies in Big Data 120,
https://doi.org/10.1007/978-981-99-3989-3_3

Technology for older people is usually verified with the same measures being used in consumer electronics usability evaluation, like usage, efficiency, reliability, and accuracy [12–17]. We believe that designing for assisting older people active living, empowerment, and aging well would require interwoven knowledge strands in the areas of collection and analysis of data, in the cognitive decline and aging trajectories and in the interaction, interface, and service design.

The authors start discussing wearable technology as all the systems that can be worn by people to emphasize, augment, and increase computational use of body presence and movement in the real world, meaning the adoption of wearable technology such as sensors, actuators, displays that might appear in mobile devices such as smartphones, smart band, and other wearable devices. This chapter wants to address the broadest possible definition of wearable technology including all the digital technologies that can collect data about human body health and action, dealing with accuracy and quality of measure on the one hand, and with user adoption, acceptance and perception of utility on the other hand.

This chapter focuses on the experiential nature of the interaction with digital technology for aging population. In particular, the chapter discusses wearable technologies from a variety of perspectives, ranging from quality of interaction, and user experience to data and information provision. The main theme emerging from the discussion is m-Health wearable technologies data quality and data measurement uncertainty and how it might be managed, presented, and provided to aging people in order to make sense of them. Visualizing uncertainty is a challenging endeavor since uncertainty is computed in reference to primary data. Thus, visualizing the uncertainty should be coupled with a comprehensive knowledge of both the primary data and the uncertainty itself. Literature currently lacks accepted methodologies for visualizing uncertainty, even if Tufte [18], Bertin [19], Ware [20], and Chambers et al. [21] provided some guidance in the general visualization theory. Their findings have been used in the literature to assess uncertainty visualizations [22] and in guidance for design.

By focusing on mobile health applications we foster a human-centered design approach to wearable technologies, bringing hardware and software specifications together with user requirements, quality of experience and long-term adoption by aging populations, whose needs, expectations, wishes, capabilities, and limitations are commonly disregarded in technology development [23].

## 2 Measurement Through Wearable Technologies

This paragraph will deal with the importance of using wearable devices, to have enhanced information from m-Health technologies. m-Health represents a powerful tool to provide enhanced support to users (e.g., through coaching solutions and notifications, feedback, self-assessment). The strength and the innovation that m-Health can bring to the health and medical market lies in the possibility of providing personalized and tailor-made coaching advice and encouragement. The use of m-Health and health-coaching brings also advantage to the user, that is able to inspect its own data and apply self-assessment strategies.

In this paragraph, a list of the wearables already existing in the market and that could be used in combination with m-Health solutions will be provided.

People are increasingly using wearable technologies during their daily life, with a particular interest in the purpose of remote monitoring: especially in this field, m-Health plays a central and settled role in the next development of healthcare and aging people [24, 25]. The definition of "m-Health" tools, where "m" is an abbreviation of "mobile," covers all the devices that can be brought literally anywhere and possibly can establish an Internet connection from multiple places; this feature implies that an m-Health user is potentially always digitally connected and therefore always reachable for communications. A broader definition of m-Health explains that "m-Health is any medical and public health practices relying on mobile devices, such as cell phones, patient monitoring systems, personal digital assistants and other wireless devices." Researcher centers, health associations, and also private companies suggest that the role of the mobile-based tools is to feed people with information [26], enable and facilitate communication, remotely monitor physiological parameters [27], and decrease the visiting frequency that patients make to healthcare professionals, especially in view of pandemic situations. m-Health applications encompass a wide range of actions that comprises sending daily text messages or telemedicine actions using mobile devices (e.g., tablet, smartphones) and mobile applications coupled or not with the related bunch of sensors (bracelets, smartwatches, or smart bands) [28, 29]. m-Health technologies are becoming also crucial to properly support the management of chronic diseases [30], by performing human-centered monitoring and to perform self-assessment of their health, reminding to take medications or appointments, fitness trackers but also including the support of health workers [31]. In fact, the gradual rise of digital technologies has given benefits to m-Health innovations and highlights that there is the need to progressively renew and develop m-Health technologies.

In terms of wearable sensors, literature so far, mainly identified four main classes of m-Health applications:

- sensors for monitoring health and well-being;
- sensors for diagnostics;
- assistive sensors;
- sensors for delivering treatments.

A device is considered wearable if it is an item that can be worn, with electronic and computing technologies, that collects or displays different types of data [32]. Nowadays, smart electronics are conventional devices that bring together wearable technologies and health operations [33]. The demand for wearable sensors in the healthcare field increases steadily for applications such as remote and long-term monitoring of patients in dwellings, especially in situations such as the COVID-19 epidemic event. In fact, smartwatches and smart band are gaining the power of helping the healthcare sector and contributing to improve occupants' well-being through a day-to-day assessment of human health. On a daily basis, most of the interest and favorable challenges for m-Health applications, that will be faced in the future, are focusing on smart trackers or smartwatches. These kinds of devices are embedded with miniaturized electronics that can be coupled with a smartphone application to daily follow the user through its wellness level, physical activity, sleep monitoring, and global health status. Advancements in wireless communication, nanotechnologies, and computational power increase the chances for miniaturization and non-obtrusive physiological measurement. Wearable technologies include also smart clothing, mainly used in sports and health territory, but recent developments are focusing on the measurement and monitoring of physiological data collected from the human body. In addition, the market of smart devices is also crowded with smart rings, smart headbands, and smart glasses to measure health-related parameters.

As an example, innovative m-Health technology is represented by smart contact lenses, produced by Google, equipped with a miniaturized sensor to measure the concentration of glucose in blood, directly from the tears of people in real-time, with the benefit of decreasing the pain of the user, taking over the conventional detection method. Smart headbands are produced with thermoelectric cooling technology to immediately cool down the embedded ice pack and effectively alleviate headaches. Earlobe miniaturized sensors that are embedded with photoplethysmography and continuous wave radar can be used to measure continuously blood pressure [34, 35]. The University of California also has produced a tattoo sticker that is able to continuously measure blood glucose and a flexible sensor that can retrieve uric acid data by placing it in the mouth [36]. Skin adhesive patches are also developed by directly coupling them with the skin, not to have high-quality and reliable assessment of many physiological and pathophysiological signals from the body, but also advertises adequate transcutaneous medical treatment with high patient acceptance and safety. Currently, the most employed adhesive patches can distribute drugs through the skin because they are an alternative to oral delivery and hypodermic injection. Skin adhesive patches are now equipped with onboard sensing system, to monitor vital parameters, thanks to recent advancements in flexible and miniaturized electronics. These devices are thin flexible patches where conducting or semiconducting nanomaterials can acquire high-quality ECG and EMG signals. Smart garments or textiles are other categories of wearable technology: in fact, smart clothing, usually an m vest or close-fitting shirt, can be provided with onboard smart sensors. As an example, smart shoes are an attractive form of smart devices: they provide accurate and flexible biomechanical analysis and can be employed to monitor gait, to automatically assess functional biomechanics (Fig. 1).

Given the above premises, there is a need to implement systems that are comfortable, easy to use, and possibly have a good design; in [37] is highlighted that the participants' preferences for home health monitoring are comfortable devices, and most of them express their willingness to use the smart band [37].

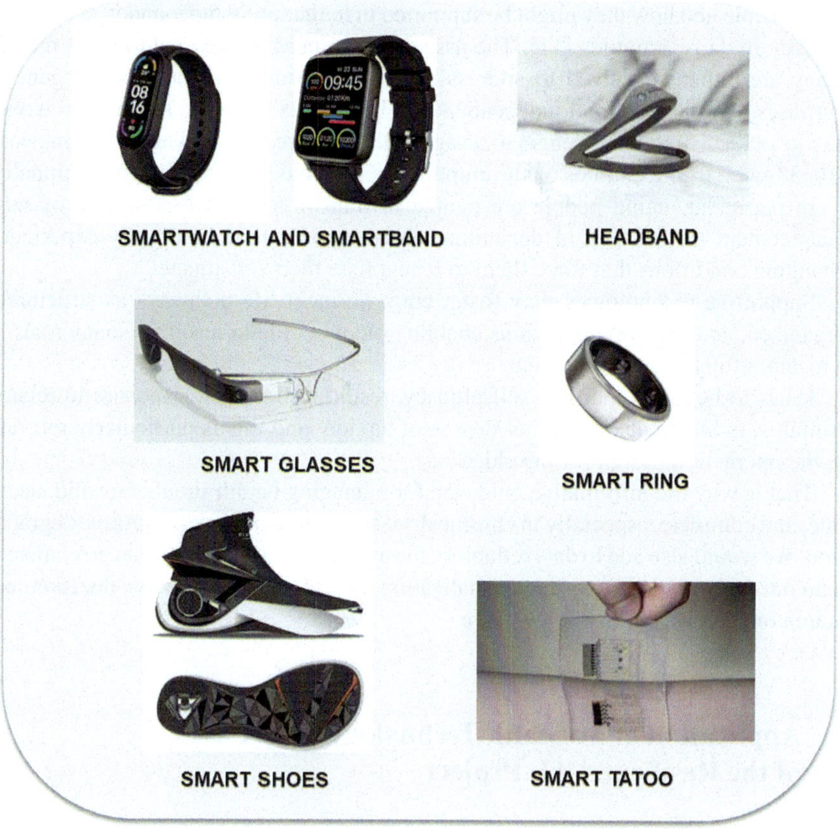


**Fig. 1** Picture of the different wearable smart devices

## 3 Aging People Experience and Informative Needs

Aging people are undergoing a dynamically changing life experience that involve from slight to major adaptations in behavior, cognition, and social relation. In particular, meanwhile older people recognize capabilities' changes over time, they also require raising their awareness of increasingly limitation of personal autonomy, care, and health self-management. As a consequence, their independence can be supported only if it is constantly renegotiated [24] through supportive and assistive technologies. In this research we want to address how positive and insightful purposes, like active lifestyle, self-caring and cognitive activation, might be pursued with a design research action, rather than focusing on tackling challenges that might be only partially solved since naturally brought by aging, such as cognitive decline and memory degradation.

In this context, Active Living is proposed as a cornerstone concept that allows the researchers to frame what does living an active and meaningful life means for older people and how they might be supported in maintaining independence and self-efficacy in daily activities [11]. The assistive systems currently sold on the market today are either conceived to address specific functionalities or to serve general purposes, like the “optimal independence” [37]. In this research, the authors would like to tackle a higher challenge: to design within the “resourceful aging” framework [10, 38] which concentrates on the empowerment of older people in aging rationally.

In particular, aging people are people in transition: from a condition of self-management to the need of depending on caregivers, they constantly experience changing conditions that force them to renegotiate their self-image.

Supportive technologies may foster empowerment life pathways as structured, organized, and goal-oriented paths enabling older people to reach personal goals in a meaningfully rich environment.

It has to be noted that low self-efficacy, resulting from few exposure to related stimulus, is linked also to higher degree of anxiety and this is particularly relevant in the interaction design for the elderly.

That is why the informative guidance for managing health should be solid, accurate, and complete, especially in chronic disease management and cognitive degradation. We would also add to data reliability the user ability to interpret data, to elaborate data into information from data visualization and, ultimately, to make decision and action on the basis of that knowledge.

## 4 Application of m-health Technology: Use Case of the Resilient AAL Project

In this paragraph, we describe the specific use case of m-Health technologies in the context of aging people and Active Living. The research is conducted using the combination of two m-Health devices: a smartwatch and a social tablet, provided with a dedicated application. The promising role of this technology for aging people is typically known, although the use of m-Health tools in prevention and health monitoring on a daily basis for seniors is still unexplored [38]. Positive changes in health-related lifestyle of seniors can provide and increase health benefits. Promoting health among this vulnerable category may give benefit for increasing life expectancy [39]. Even if it is well-known the importance of a healthy lifestyle, seniors (50+ years) are very often physically inactive. But to what extent is the use of such tools by older adults reported in the literature?

The decline of pathologies or early diagnosis are typical examples of applications of the Active and Assisted Living (AAL) field [24]; moreover, remote monitoring of seniors affected by Mild Cognitive Impairment (MCI) in combination with proper data analysis techniques permits to detect long-term modifications of the disease and related health service [40, 41].

Within this framework, the RESILIEN-T project (Technology driven self-management for building resilience among people with early-stage cognitive impairment, AAL Program) is involved in the development of a new and customizable ICT platform for the autonomous monitoring and administration of seniors' affected by mild cognitive impairment (MCI), to build up the self-monitoring skill of seniors, in order to decelerate the behavioral decline.

The ratio behind the project is that a mixed solution of two or more devices, already on the market (i.e., social tablet for seniors, lifestyle monitoring systems, wearables) and additional software development (e.g., mobile app or cloud systems) will help MCI-affected people to self-monitor their status. The RESILIEN-T system considered as use case in this research is an ICT solution made of a social tablet and smartwatch for monitoring physical activity and other physiological parameters of the senior.

The RESILIEN-T platform is modular and interoperable and is centered around a tablet to gather data from the different version of the system. The tablet sends the collected data through the dedicated API, to the Cloud, in which data are saved and used for further processing. Formal and informal carees can access this data from the dedicated applications.

The seniors recruited to test the RESILIEN-T platform participated in a measurement campaign that implied the daily use of the smartwatch that was daily collecting specific data. The campaign had the scope of defining a measurement set-up, procedure, and data analysis to deliver coaching advice to MCI-affected seniors to coach them on how to maintain a healthy and active life. To this aim, this research is focused on the Plus version of RESILIEN-T platform, to develop dedicated algorithms, based on the quantities measured by the smartwatch and evaluating the impact of the measurement uncertainty of the measured quantities, in the feedback provided to the user through the m-Health application. The output of the algorithm is to classify the data collected from the smartwatch, into three categories that represent whether the user exhibits a normal or abnormal behavior.

## 5 The Problem of the Measurement Uncertainty

The International Vocabulary of Metrology defines the measurement uncertainty as a "parameter characterizing the dispersion of the quantity values being attributed to a measure" that describes the interval where the value of the measured parameter is assumed to lie, with a stated level of confidence. On the basis of this definition, the concept of measurement uncertainty can be applied to the quantity measured by commercial smartwatches: m-Health leans on the measurement of quantities, which are derived from the processing of signal coming from embedded sensors, e.g., accelerometer, that should be characterized from a metrological point of view. Therefore, if the measured quantities are evaluated and measured with the final aim of providing coaching solutions to the end-user, we should quantify if the measurement uncertainty has an impact on this process.

At this scope, the use case is about the Plus version of RESILIEN-T, in which a tailored routine, based on a statistical analysis was developed, using the quantities collected by a commercial smartwatch. As stated, the output of this algorithm is subjected to a measurement uncertainty, due to the intrinsic characteristics of the smartwatch, that should be quantified. The algorithm has the final scope of classifying the behavior of seniors, expressed by the data collected by the smartwatch, by classifying the data in "Normality," "Negative Abnormality" or "Positive Abnormality," to deliver custom-made coaching advice according to the output of the classification. The results of this classification are used for the decision-making process to create customized coaching task to promote health living and active life.

The identified problem is that when using wearable devices in m-Health, the sensors installed on the devices are used to extract raw data, which is processed by the device's processor, to derive more complex quantities. A practical example, which is mainly the focus of this chapter, can be found starting from the data of the accelerometer, a sensor increasingly present in wearable devices. The accelerometric data are useful for the extraction of further parameters, such as, for example, the number of steps performed by the user, the calories consumed during the day, the distance traveled, etc. In a metrological context, the number of steps is a derived quantity, and it is therefore important to define the measurement uncertainty of this quantity. Typically, producers of commercial smart band and smartwatches do not provide in their datasheet the measurement uncertainty of the derived quantities. Therefore, in the case of the number of steps, researchers typically perform ad-hoc experiments to estimate the measurement uncertainty of the wearable device, against a reference method. Next section will describe in detail the procedure applied.

## 5.1 Applied Methodology

The authors selected the wearable activity tracker iHealth Wave watch (HW) (iHealth Lab Inc.). The parameters that are daily monitored by the device are: daily steps (counts), distance traveled (km), calories burned (kcal), sleep efficiency (%), and the time spent in the bed (hh:mm). The wearable is equipped with a 3-axis accelerometer that can monitor physical activities. Raw data from the sensors are processed in the Cloud.

Two participants were involved in this use case, one male and one female (User 1 and User 2, respectively). User 1 is 70 years old, while User 2 is 63 years old; they live together, and do not suffer from any pathology, so they can perform physical activities daily. The two users provided this information by filling in a dedicated questionnaire, completed after signing the informed consent, which described the purpose of the research. The smartwatch was given to each participant for five months after signing informed consent about the purpose of the study, according to the Declaration of Helsinki, in compliance with the Guidelines for Good Clinical Practice. It is important to underline that the proposed research is not a clinical trial and that the data provided by the smartwatch are fully anonymized. The proposed methodology is observational and collected data were used with the aim of defining an operational procedure. Data were collected from October 2020 to February 2021. The developed methodology is summarized in Fig. 2.

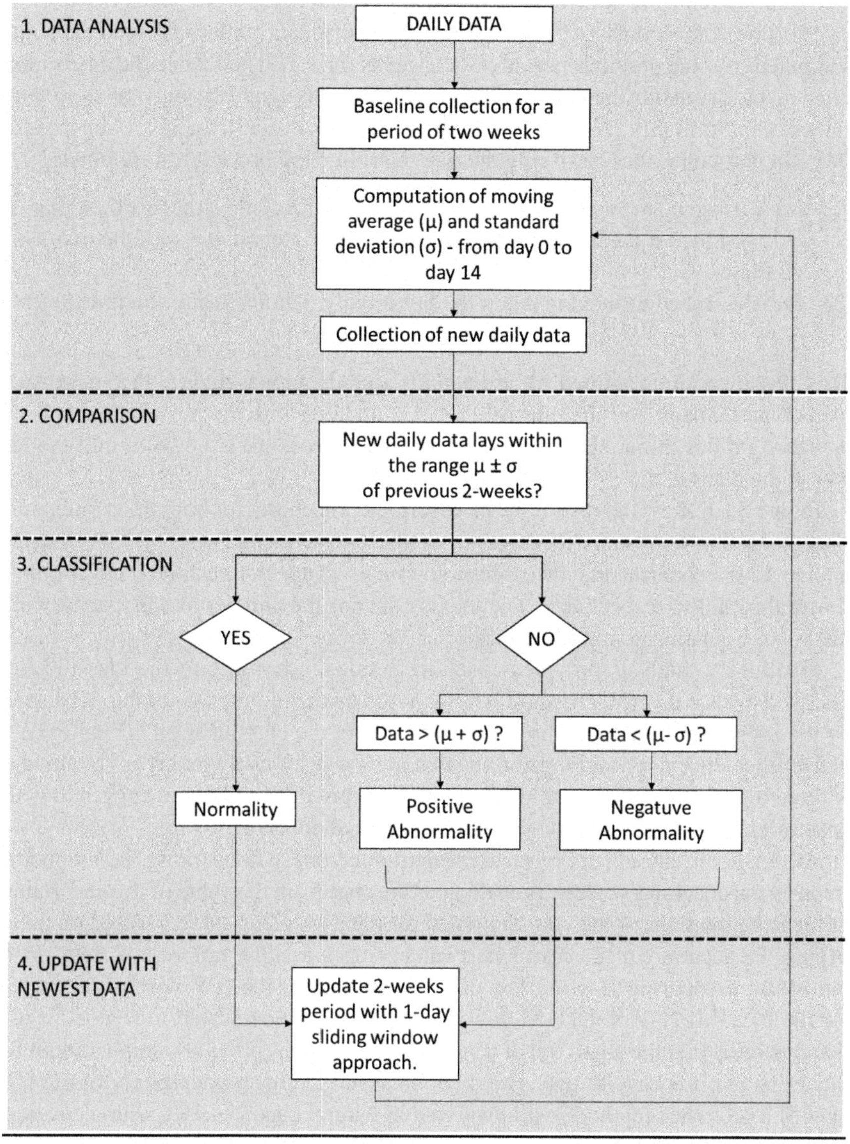


**Fig. 2** Description of the overall algorithm used to classify the behavior of users that wears the iHealth smartwatch. The described procedure is applied for the number of daily steps collected from the smartwatch

The first step of the algorithm consisted of the collection of the baseline data that comprises collected data over a period of two weeks; this data will build up the baseline. The following step is the assessment of the moving average ($m$) and standard deviation ($s$), calculated for a period of two weeks, chosen after visually investigating the data, according to the state of the art [42].

The procedure consists of comparing the daily data with a pre-defined range computed over the previous period of two weeks ($m \pm s$). Then, once the day is identified inside or outside the proposed range, the day is assigned to one of the following categories: Normality (*N*), Positive Abnormality (*PA*), and Negative Abnormality (*NA*). In particular, for classifying the day the following procedure is applied:

(1) *NA* is assigned to the day when the latest daily data is below the threshold ($m-s$).
(2) *N* is assigned if the latest daily data is inside the interval $m \pm s$ of the two-week baseline.
(3) *PA* is assigned to the day when the latest daily data is greater the threshold ($m + s$).

This classification is applied for every daily step data measured by the smartwatch of each participant, and the interval $m \pm s$ is updated with the moving average and the standard deviation, shifting of one day. The procedure is iterated until the last day of the dataset.

Figure 3a, b show the results of the described procedure, for both the participants. The green line represents the average of the two-week interval, and the red and orange lines represent the two thresholds $m + s$ (upper threshold) and the $m-s$ (lower threshold), respectively. The y-axis contains the number of daily steps, while the x-axis contains the monitored days.

Finally, the analysis provides coaching actions, according to the classification assigned to each day (*N*, *PA*, and *NA*). So, based on the monitoring of the steps made by the user daily, measured through the wearable, the classification is employed to deliver thee different coaching actions that are suggestions if the day is classified as *N*, greetings and compliments when the day is classified as *PA* and suggestions for promoting physical activity when the day is classified as *NA*.

At this point, the impact of measurement uncertainty in counting the number of steps on the coaching strategy is evaluated. We start from the value of the uncertainty of measurement: the value was computed during a previous study focused on quantifying the accuracy of a set of smartwatches on measured number of steps. With this study, comparing also the low cost of this device, the HW watch was chosen for the RESILIEN-T project. Moreover, in a workshop dedicated to seniors, it was demonstrated that the smartwatch is approved because it provides simple output for the users and it is easy to use. The computed measurement uncertainty of the HW against a reference method, while walking at natural pace is 4.7%, with a coverage factor k equal to 2 [43]. This result means that the dispersion of the quantity values being attributed to the read value of the step measurement is 4.7%, which means that the read value lies within the range ± 4.7%. In particular, Fig. 4a shows the daily trend of the number of steps measured from User 1, with the related interval due to

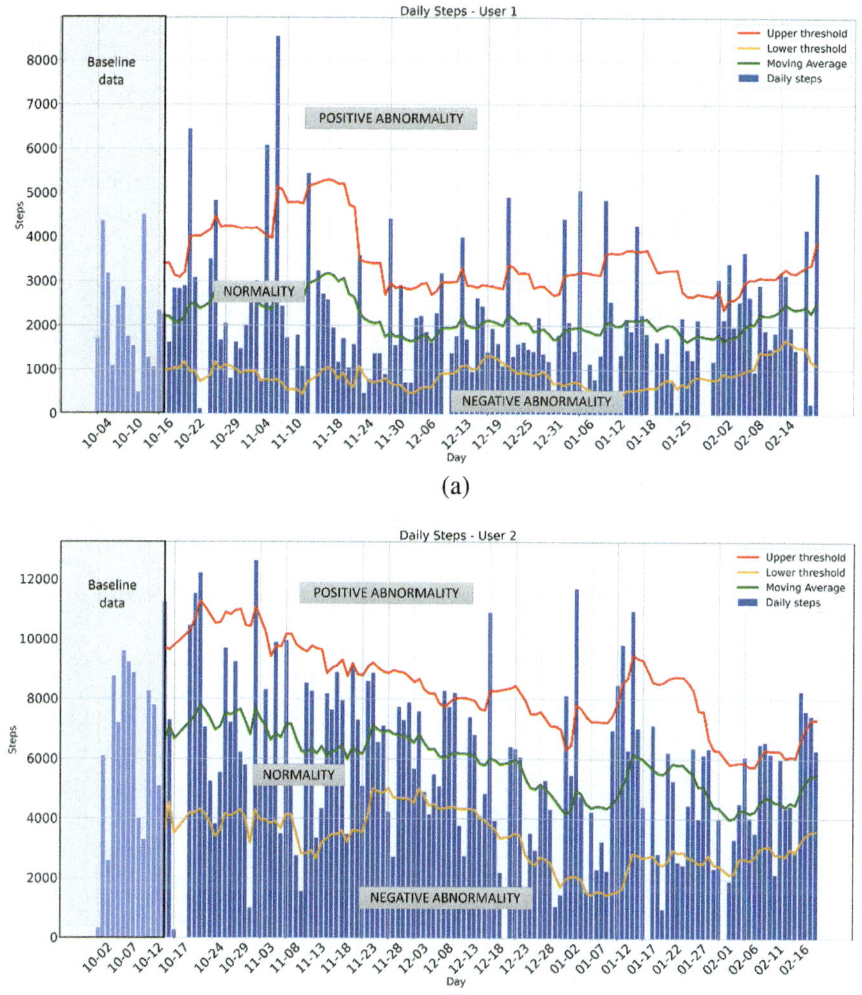


(a)

(b)

**Fig. 3** Example of the collected data for User 1 (**a**) and User 2 (**b**) and the related computed $m$ and $s$

the measurement uncertainty (black line), which comprises the set of values that can be attributed to the measured number of steps.

Figure 4b illustrates more clearly the definition of "uncertain" day, which in this case is defined when the measured number of steps and the related interval due to the measurement uncertainty (in this case $\pm$ 4.7%.), lie both inside and outside the range $\mu \pm \sigma$.

The number of uncertain days is computed by detecting the samples that belong to two classifications after the application of the measurement uncertainty. The number of uncertain days over the total number of days of monitoring gives the percentage of

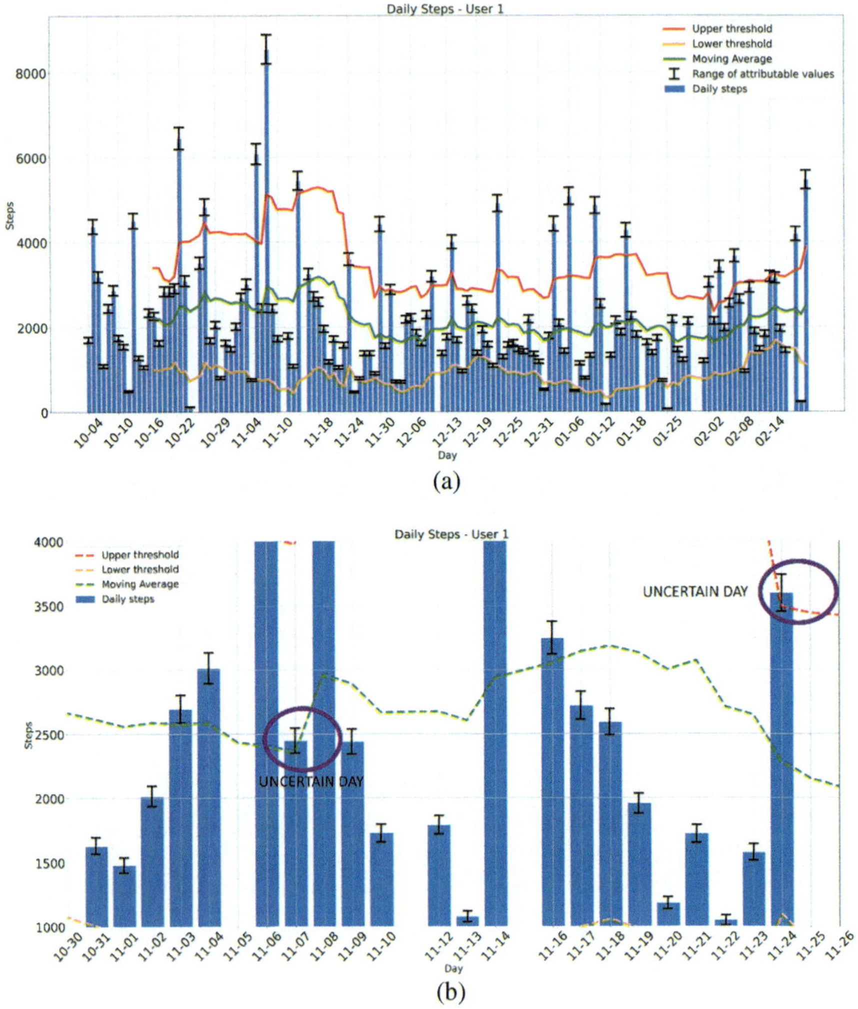


**Fig. 4** Collected step data and application of the measurement uncertainty for User 1 (**a**) and zoomed plot to display two examples of uncertain days, circled in violet, considering a measurement uncertainty of $\pm$ 4.7% (**b**)

uncertain days that could negatively impact the final purpose of providing coaching advice. By applying this procedure, it is computed that the number of days that, considering the measurement uncertainty of the device, belong to two categories, is 14, which is 11% on the total period of monitoring for User 1; for User 2, the percentage of uncertain days is 27%.

## 5.2 Predictive Models: Monte Carlo Simulation on Step Data

This paragraph will explore the possibility of using Monte Carlo simulation, to evaluate the measurement uncertainty of the number of steps, on the definition of the "Normality," "Positive Abnormality," and "Negative Abnormality" condition. A preliminary assumption is that every sensor is associated with its related measurement uncertainty; therefore, it is crucial to add how this uncertainty, associated with each parameter, affects the final measurement in the process. The Guide to the expression of uncertainty in measurement (GUM) explains the steps to compute the measurement uncertainty. Typically, this process is based on the law of propagation of uncertainties, but in case of relationships that are non-linear, the GUM suggests to evaluate the measurement uncertainty by applying the Monte Carlo method (MCM). MCM can be employed whenever the exact mathematical equation among quantities is unknown and there is no linear relationship between the input parameters. The necessary actions to apply MCM are exposed in the GUM. In general, MCM is able to give a numerical approximation of the cumulative density function (pdf) of an output quantity obtained by the relationship $y = f(x)$. The basic idea behind MCM is that each sample, $x_{i,}$ of the input parameter, should originate from a predetermined distribution; from the pdf, it is possible to extract a random sample of each input parameter $x_i$ to assess an estimation of the output quantity ($y$) and the related measurement uncertainty. Hereby, a summary of the steps taken for the purpose of this study:

- Firstly, the number of MCM trials should be chosen: in this case this quantity is chosen to be 200,000, to guarantee the 95% of coverage interval, as reported in the GUM supplement.
- A number of vectors equal to the number of MCM trials is generated. This process is done by randomly selecting a sample of the input quantity (number of steps) from the pdf, to get an ensemble of input vectors that can be used to obtain the output quantity (number of uncertain days). To extract the random sample, a Gaussian distribution, with the following simulated uncertainties 4%, 10%, 20%, 30%, 50% were created.
- Every random sample obtained is used to compute the related output quantity $y$ (number of days with uncertain category), yielding to a number of output quantity equal to the number of MCM trials.
- Previous step is used to compute the measurement uncertainty of the uncertain day.

An example of the results that can arise from the application of the measurement uncertainty is displayed in Fig. 5a, which shows the daily number of steps and the related interval of possible attributable values, when a 30% of measurement uncertainty is considered; similarly, to Figs. 4b, and 5b shows that the attributable value to the measured number of steps is wider and in turn the number of uncertain days increases.

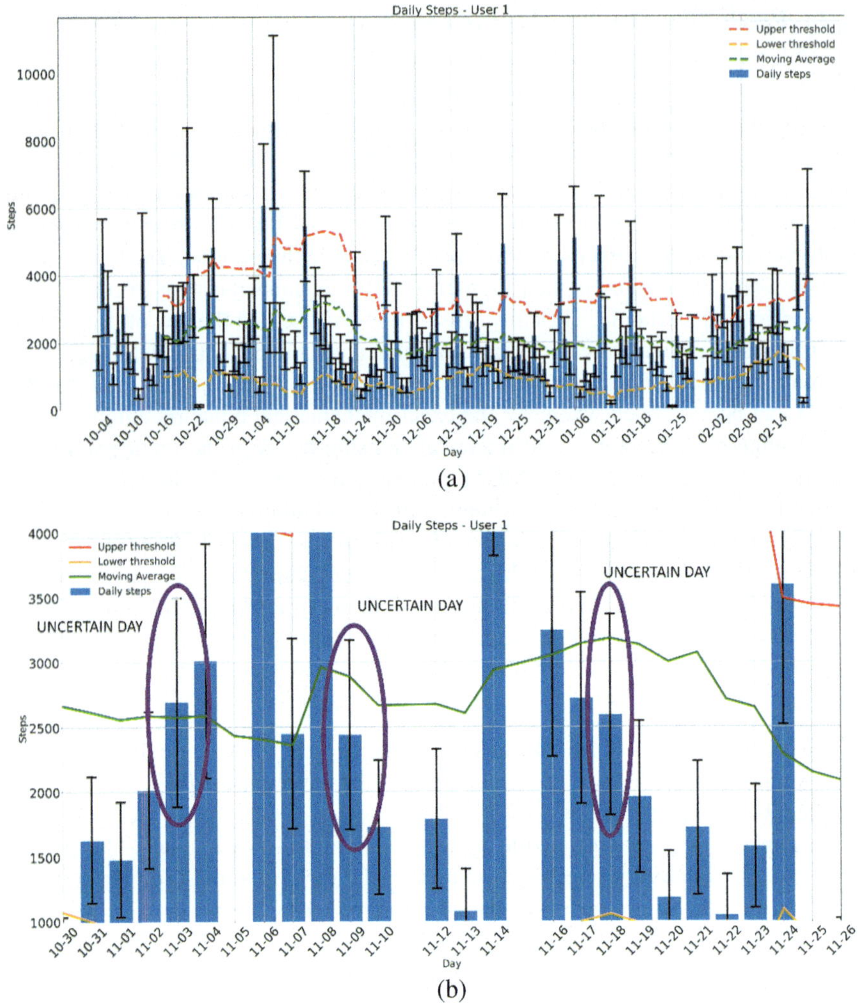


**Fig. 5** Collected step data and application of the measurement uncertainty for User 1 (**a**) and example of uncertain day by applying a measurement uncertainty of 30% (**b**)

Table 1 contains the result of the Monte Carlo simulation, which has provided the number of uncertain days due to the simulated measurement uncertainty applied to the measured number of steps. For the period of monitoring considered in this study, the number of uncertain days ranges from 5 to 37% and to 11% to 85% for User 1 and User 2 respectively and for measurement uncertainty of 4% and 50%.

There is a linear relationship (Fig. 6a, b) between the percentage of uncertain days and the measurement uncertainty, both for User 1 and User 2. The results are even more justified by the values of $R^2$ which is 0.99 both for User 1 and User 2, which expresses the goodness of the linear fit.

**Table 1** Result of the Monte Carlo simulation. The % of uncertain days is computed, according to the measurement uncertainty of the device for use User 1

| Simulated measurement uncertainty | Uncertain days | | Standard deviation | | % of Uncertain days | |
|---|---|---|---|---|---|---|
| [%] | Counts | | Counts | | [%] | |
| | User 1 | User 2 | User 1 | User 2 | User 1 | User 2 |
| **4** | 14 | 7 | 4 | 2 | 11 | 5 |
| **10** | 31 | 17 | 5 | 3 | 24 | 13 |
| **20** | 56 | 33 | 5 | 4 | 42 | 24 |
| **30** | 78 | 50 | 5 | 5 | 59 | 37 |
| **50** | 113 | 84 | 6 | 5 | 85 | 61 |

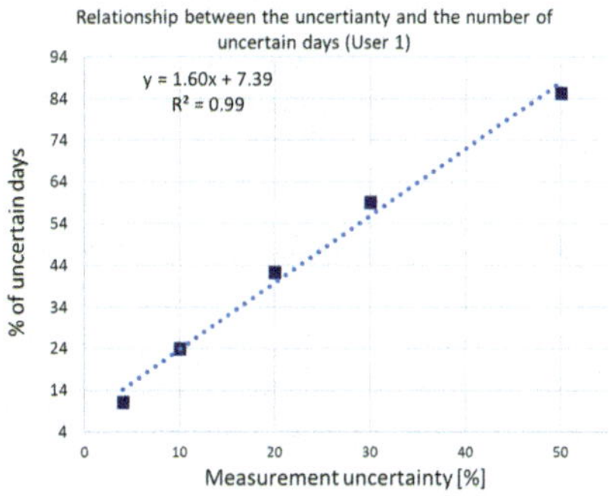


(a)

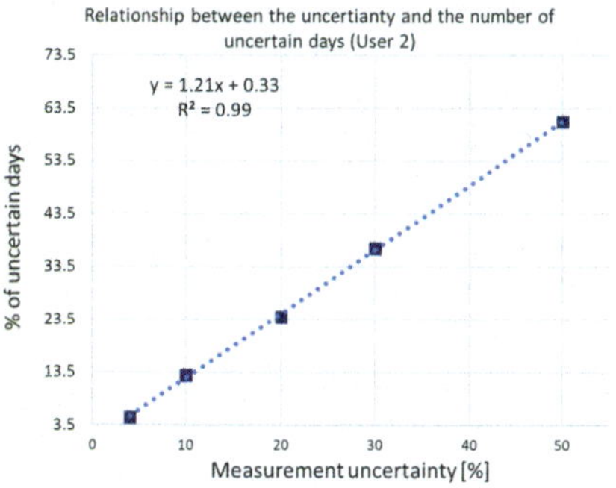


(b)

**Fig. 6** Relationship between the simulated measurement uncertainty and the corresponding number of uncertain days computed through Monte Carlo simulation for User 1 (**a**) and User 2 (**b**)

# 6 Conclusion

Literature analysis has recognized the role of m-Health technologies in promoting healthy lifestyle for older people. Furthermore, the m-Health technology might be used to preserve, and if possible, to enrich social companionship by connecting people with relatives and friends also during social distancing and isolation. Understanding uncertainty in m-Health not only impacts the interpretation of medical data and healthcare but on attitude, knowledge and behavior of the aging population. And that makes it critical for technologists to design and implement monitoring and coaching interactive systems, as in the RESILIEN-T project. This case allows us to summarize some guiding principles to further develop this domain from both an empirical and a theoretical perspective.

When presenting the source of the data, visualization designers may associate uncertain information, for example, in the form of a range of error. But we wonder what the impact of visualizing uncertainty is and if this is mostly a matter for expert's professionals and researchers able to appreciate "exact" visualizations of uncertainty information [44].

At the same time, we consider that the target panel of aging people doesn't have the competence, the expectation, and the objective of uncertainty interpretation. What counts for them is the decision they can make upon certain information: what is the data, what does communicate to them and, ultimately, what's the suggestion for their ordinary life. With reference to the framework for uncertainty communication [45, 46], we might take the characteristics of the audiences as fundamental requirements for the design, for example, in terms of the different levels of graphical literacy and their ability to disentangle complex visualizations. In particular, the consequences of this design must be evaluated: do their proposition provoke uncomfortable emotional responses or, even worst, rejection of the application. Indeed, interface information visualizations are among the key aspects that allow to build credibility and trust in the system.

The authors have discussed measurement issues in the RESILIEN-T case, and how uncertainty measurements might be used to provide coaching advice to promote a healthy and active life. Classification strategies (such as Normality, Positive Abnormality, Positive Normality) can deliver suggestions, congratulations, or demand for more physical activity and in case have been implemented to foster trust of technology and, ultimately, aging people's acceptance and adoption. That is why an important effort has to be made by designers on expressing the measurement uncertainty [45], the layout of the uncertainty communication, in terms of indicators, or visualizations, the way of communicating, such as print, online, broadcast, or verbal conversation.

Authors' viewpoints from different perspectives give an empirical comprehension of uncertainty issues and how they relate to interaction design for elderly people. If the uncertainty of data needs to be mastered by designers and engineers in implementing ICT for elderly people, e.g., the number of uncertain days over the total number, the visualization of uncertainty is what provokes an impact on the final meaning of coaching advice. Indeed, the factors relating to what effect the communication has on the audience cognition, emotion, trust, and behavior and decision-making are of predominant importance. If the research on uncertainty visualization and measurement [47] has identified popular techniques accompanied by their merits and shortcomings the effects of uncertainty communication on acceptance; trust and adoption of technology and, eventually, behavioral change still need to be investigated in the context of active living of aging population.

## References

1. Nielsen, J.: Usability Engineering. Morgan Kaufmann (1994)
2. Nielsen, J.: Ten Usability Heuristics (2005)

3. Fisk, A.D., Czaja, S.J., Rogers, W.A., Charness, N., Sharit, J.: Designing for older adults: principles and creative human factors approaches second edition. In: Designing for Older Adults, pp. 1–232. Taylor and Francis (2009)
4. Kline, D.W.: Aging effects on Vision: impairment, variability, self-report and compensatory change. In: Schaie, K.W., Charness, N. (eds.) Impact of Technology on Successful Aging, pp. 85–99. Springer, New York (2003)
5. Morrell, R.W., Holt, B.J., Dailey, S.R., Feldman, C., Mayhorn, C.B., Echt, K.V., Podany, K.I.: Older Adults and Information Technology: A Compendium of Scientific Research and Web Site Accessibility Guidelines. National Institute on Aging, Washington (2001)
6. Hawthorn, D.: Possible implications of aging for interface designers. Interact. Comput. **12**, 507–528 (2000)
7. Schieber, F.: Human factors and aging: Identifying and compensating for age-related deficits in sensory and cognitive function. In: Schaie, K.W., Charness, N. (eds.) Influences of Technological Change on Individual Aging, pp. 42–84. Springer (2003)
8. Giaccardi, E., Kuijer, L., Neven, L.: Design for resourceful ageing : intervening in the ethics of gerontechnology: 2016 Design Research Society Conference (DRS 2016. In: Proceedings of DRS 2016, Design + Research + Society Future-Future-Focused Thinking, vol. 1, June 27–30. Brighton, UK (2016)
9. Antonietti, A., Balconi, M., Catellani, P., Marchetti, A.: Empowering skills for an active ageing and healthy living. In: Active Ageing and Healthy Living, pp. 157–171 (2014) https://doi.org/10.3233/978-1-61499-425-1-157
10. Sellen, A., Rogers, Y., Harper, R., Rodden, T.: Reflecting human values in the digital age. Assoc. Comput. Mach. **52**, 58–66 (2009). https://doi.org/10.1145/1467247.1467265
11. Social Exclusion and Information and Communication Technologies: Lessons from Studies of Single Parents and the Young Elderly—Leslie Haddon (2000). https://journals.sagepub.com/doi/abs/10.1177/14614448000002004001
12. Czaja, S.J., et al.: Factors predicting the use of technology: Findings from the center for research and education on aging and technology enhancement (create). Psychol. Aging **21**, 333–352 (2006)
13. Hernández-Encuentra, E., Pousada, M., Gómez-Zúñiga, B.: ICT and older people: beyond usability. Educ. Gerontol. **35**, 226–245 (2009)
14. Mitzner, T.L., et al.: Older adults talk technology: technology usage and attitudes. Comput. Hum. Behav. **26**, 1710–1721 (2010)
15. O'Brien, M.A., Olson, K.E., Charness, N., Czaja, S.J., Fisk, A.D., Rogers, W.A., Sharit, J.: Understanding technology usage in older adults. In: Proceedings of the 6th International Society for Gerontechnology, pp. 1–5. Pisa (2008)
16. Olson, K.E., O'Brien, M.A., Rogers, W.A., Charness, N.: Diffusion of technology: frequency of use for younger and older adults. Ageing Int. **36**, 123–145 (2011)
17. Reddy, G.R., Blackler, A., Popovic, V.: Adaptable interface framework for intuitively learnable product interfaces for people with diverse capabilities. In: Intuitive Interaction. CRC Press (2018)
18. Tufte, E.R.: The visual display of quantitative information. J. Healthc. Quality (JHQ) **7**, 15 (1985)
19. Bertin, J.: Semiology of Graphics. The University of Wisconsin Press, Madison, Wisconsin (1983)
20. Ware, C.: Information Visualization: Perception for Design. Morgan Kaufmann (2019)
21. Chambers, J.M., Cleveland, W.S., Kleiner, B., Tukey, P.A.: Graphical Methods for Data Analysis. Chapman and Hall/CRC (2017). https://doi.org/10.1201/9781351072304
22. Riveiro, M.: Evaluation of uncertainty visualization techniques for information fusion. In: 2007 10th International Conference on Information Fusion, pp. 1–8 (2007). https://doi.org/10.1109/ICIF.2007.4408049
23. Pollini, A., Giacobone, G.A., Zannoni, M.: Aging and interaction: designing for active living experiences. In: Scataglini, S., Imbesi, S., Marques, G. (eds.) Internet of Things for Human-Centered Design: Application to Elderly Healthcare, pp. 39–61. Springer Nature (2022). https://doi.org/10.1007/978-981-16-8488-3_3

24. Casaccia, S., Revel, G.M., Scalise, L.: AI-based sensor network for ADLs monitoring on ageing people during COVID-19 epidemic. In: 2021 IEEE International Workshop on Metrology for Industry 4.0 IoT (MetroInd4.0 IoT), pp. 290–294 (2021). https://doi.org/10.1109/MetroInd4.0IoT51437.2021.9488438
25. Norris, A.C., Stockdale, R.S., Sharma, S.: A strategic approach to m-health. Health Inf. J. **15**, 244–253 (2009)
26. Application of mobile health to support the elderly during the COVID-19 outbreak: a systematic review—ScienceDirect. https://www.sciencedirect.com/science/article/pii/S2211883722000016?casa_token=NFdPhkvbamEAAAAA:xQc0fNLYcV4flXQpffBeyqhKdaogvYsVdmO-2wKC554Lkkx7rxdhdwEvApZY78lUeR-Z3oP0
27. Beltrán-Chávez, F., et al.: Chapter 14 - M-health system for cardiac and COVID patient monitoring using body sensor networks and machine learning. In: de Pablos, P.O., Chui, K.T., Lytras, M.D. (eds.) Digital Innovation for Healthcare in COVID-19 Pandemic, pp. 217–244. Academic Press (2022). https://doi.org/10.1016/B978-0-12-821318-6.00011-6
28. Evaluation of Mobile Health apps for Non-Medical Cannabis Use: A Scoping Review—ScienceDirect. https://www.sciencedirect.com/science/article/pii/S1877050921022754
29. Park, S., et al.: Medication event monitoring system for infectious tuberculosis treatment in Morocco: a retrospective cohort study. Int. J. Environ. Res. Public Health **16**, 412 (2019)
30. Park, H.S., Cho, H., Kim, H.S.: Development of a multi-agent m-Health application based on various protocols for chronic disease self-management. J Med. Syst. **40**, 36 (2015)
31. Free, C., et al.: The effectiveness of M-health technologies for improving health and health services: a systematic review protocol. BMC. Res. Notes **3**, 250 (2010)
32. Casaccia, S., Revel, G.M., Cosoli, G., Scalise, L.: Assessment of domestic well-being: from perception to measurement. IEEE Instrum. Meas. Mag. **24**, 58–67 (2021)
33. Rai, A., et al.: Smart sensors transforms healthcare system. In: Deep Learning and IoT in Healthcare Systems: Paradigms and Applications (2021)
34. Wearable and Biocompatible Blood Oxygen Sensor Based on Heterogeneously Integrated Lasers on a Laser-Induced Graphene Electrode | ACS Applied Electronic Materials. https://pubs.acs.org/doi/full/10.1021/acsaelm.1c01269
35. Pour Ebrahim, M., et al.: Blood pressure estimation using on-body continuous wave Radar and photoplethysmogram in various posture and exercise conditions. Sci. Rep. **9**, 16346 (2019)
36. Ramya, K., Indu, A., Akhila, B., Aswini, G., Babu, P.B.: Blood glucose monitoring techniques 7
37. Rochmawati, E., Kamilah, F., Iskandar, A.C.: Acceptance of e-health technology among older people: a qualitative study. Nurs. Health Sci. **24**, 437–446 (2022)
38. Grossman, J.T., Frumkin, M.R., Rodebaugh, T.L., Lenze, E.J.: mHealth assessment and intervention of depression and anxiety in older adults. Harv Rev Psychiatry **28**, 203–214 (2020)
39. Pronk, N., et al.: Promoting health and well-being in healthy people 2030. J. Public Health Manag. Pract. **27**, S242–S248 (2021)
40. Bevilacqua, R., et al.: Coaching through technology: a systematic review into efficacy and effectiveness for the ageing population. Int. J. Environ. Res. Public Health **17**, 5930 (2020)
41. Casaccia, S., et al.: Assistive sensor-based technology driven self-management for building resilience among people with early stage cognitive impairment. In: 2019 IEEE International Symposium on Measurements & Networking (M&N), pp. 1–5 (2019). https://doi.org/10.1109/IWMN.2019.8804998
42. Mitchell, M., Lau, E., White, L., Faulkner, G.: Commercial app use linked with sustained physical activity in two Canadian provinces: a 12-month quasi-experimental study. Int. J. Behav. Nutr. Phys. Act. **17**, 24 (2020)
43. Arpaia, P., Callegaro, L., Cultrera, A., Esposito, A. Ortolano, M.: Metrological characterization of a low-cost electroencephalograph for wearable neural interfaces in industry 4.0 applications. In: 2021 IEEE International Workshop on Metrology for Industry 4.0 IoT (MetroInd4.0 IoT), pp. 1–5 (2021). https://doi.org/10.1109/MetroInd4.0IoT51437.2021.9488445
44. Brodlie, K., Allendes Osorio, R., Lopes, A.A.: Review of uncertainty in data visualization. In: Dill, J., Earnshaw, R., Kasik, D., Vince, J., Wong, P.C. (eds.) Expanding the Frontiers of

Visual Analytics and Visualization, pp. 81–109. Springer (2012). https://doi.org/10.1007/978-1-4471-2804-5_6
45. Communicating uncertainty about facts, numbers and science | Royal Society Open Science. https://royalsocietypublishing.org/doi/full/10.1098/rsos.181870
46. Lasswell, H.D.: The structure and function of communication in society 14
47. Kamal, A., et al.: Recent advances and challenges in uncertainty visualization: a survey. J. Vis. **24**, 861–890 (2021)

# Digital Twins and Healthcare: Quick Overview and Human-Centric Perspectives

**Giacinto Barresi, Andrea Gaggioli, Federico Sternini, Alice Ravizza, Claudio Pacchierotti, and Lorenzo De Michieli**

## 1 Introduction

Emulating and simulating complex systems are computational strategies [1] for understanding phenomena that could difficultly be investigated through traditional approaches based on experiments. Emulating a system implies that a behavior is replicated without necessarily modeling its internal state. Simulations typically also include a model of the inner structure and functioning of a system: through its output, a simulation can be used for validating such an internal model. Following and transcending these approaches, recent technologies called Digital Twins have emerged over the past few years in multiple domains—from robotic manufacturing to precision medicine [2–6]. The versatility of these solutions is accompanied by the impressive efforts in exploring their capabilities of predicting future states of complex systems through a (possibly) bidirectional real-time data flow. Such features are enabled by pervasive sensor networks (as in Internet of Things, IoT), advanced visualization

G. Barresi (✉) · L. De Michieli
Rehab Technologies Lab, Istituto Italiano di Tecnologia (IIT), Genova, Italy
e-mail: giacinto.barresi@iit.it

A. Gaggioli
Research Center in Communication Psychology, Università Cattolica del Sacro Cuore, Milan, Italy

Applied Technology for Neuro-Psychology Lab, IRCCS Istituto Auxologico Italiano, Milan, Italy

F. Sternini · A. Ravizza
USE-ME-D srl, I3P Politecnico di Torino, Torino, Italy

F. Sternini
PolitoBIOMed Lab, Politecnico di Torino, Torino, Italy

C. Pacchierotti
CNRS, Univ Rennes, Inria, IRISA, Rennes, France



S. Scataglini et al. (eds.), *mHealth and Human-Centered Design Towards Enhanced Health, Care, and Well-Being*, Studies in Big Data 120,
https://doi.org/10.1007/978-981-99-3989-3_4

options (like the various extended reality items), and high-performance infrastructures (as the 5G/6G) alongside big data analytics solutions (supported by systems for Artificial Intelligence, AI) [7, 8].

This promising approach is described in this chapter before focusing on its health-related applications [9]: indeed, major initiatives in research are facing the challenge of replicating biological systems—in particular, biological agents or their organs—or the systems that include them (a setting like a home, a hospital, a city). The goal of developing Digital Twins in biomedical domains is obviously the improvement of our ways to understand and manage health issues and healthcare services (especially in terms of sustainability), and it is still in its childhood, often in research laboratories.

However, major issues must be discussed to appropriately handle the development of these (sometime) futuristic solutions, in particular when current technologies (as in Internet of Medical Things—IoMT—and mobile Health—mHealth) seem ready to bring them to us for promoting a change in our behaviors for self-care. This chapter will dedicate a section to two human-centric sub-topics—specifically: the Phygital Twins as intuitive solutions to explore a phenomenon, the ethical issues in twinning procedures and results. These constitute examples of potential next steps in making this domain grow without ignoring the human requirements. These topics are just examples of the challenges that must be faced for developing these technologies that promise to revolutionize our healthcare approaches.

## 2 Digital Twins

The recent intensive exploration of Digital Twins as data-intensive network-based computational systems is surely supported by cutting-edge advances in several domains, including data collection (environmental and wearable sensors, IoT systems), data processing (AI, systems for machine learning and deep learning, solutions for big data analytics), and data visualization with interactive features (virtual reality, various types of augmented reality and mixed reality, and, in general, the whole class of extended reality solutions). In general, Digital Twins exploit these solutions to manage the challenges (e.g., sustainability) of complex and unpredictable systems in real world, from cells to Smart Cities [10–17]. Considering its most typical definitions, a Digital Twin needs a real-time connection between a set of items in the real world and their counterparts in a virtual world, based on data about the first and their multimodal computational representations. Even if the common goal of the Digital Twins implementation is to monitor, predict, and manage uncertain conditions in complex systems [18], their heterogeneous applications and integration levels make difficult to generally agree on one definition for this class of technologies. Furthermore, a Digital Twin can model a real item like a structural or functional component, an asset, a system, a process: such a variety of representational levels affects the definition of Digital Twins with additional multiplicity. An analysis of this concept history (including the 2012 NASA roadmap about information technology and processing with focus on modeling and simulation) is beyond the scope of this chapter and can be performed according to reviews like [19–23].

However, Fuller et al. [24] proficiently handled the task of describing Digital Twins (Fig. 1) and their applied domains, as discussed in [25]. The authors highlighted how a Digital Twin is not a mere offline digital model that simulates a physical object (the Physical Twin). It must also be highlighted how a Digital Twin cannot be reduced to a digital shadow, which depicts a physical object and automatically adjusts its structure to it, while the Physical Twin can just be manually modified. According to the authors, a virtual system replicating a physical system should be fully labeled as a Digital Twin if its changes automatically replicate and influence the conditions of its Physical Twin. In such a case, we can acknowledge the bidirectional flow of data between digital and physical items of the twinning process [26]. Moreover, [27] considers the Digital Twin as an adaptive virtual model emulating the behavior of a physical system according to real-time data.

Through these features, the Digital Twin can be "played" by humans with specific expertise and decision-making roles (e.g., managers, engineers, designers) as an interactive simulation enabling the prediction of future issues in the real world based on past and current states and behaviors of the Physical Twin. This can lead to improve and optimize the physical system through interventions on policies and decision-making processes of experts evaluating the Digital Twin. According to literature analyzed in [28], it is possible to define a taxonomy of Digital Twins based on the features frequently occurring in most papers on this topic. For instance, the Physical

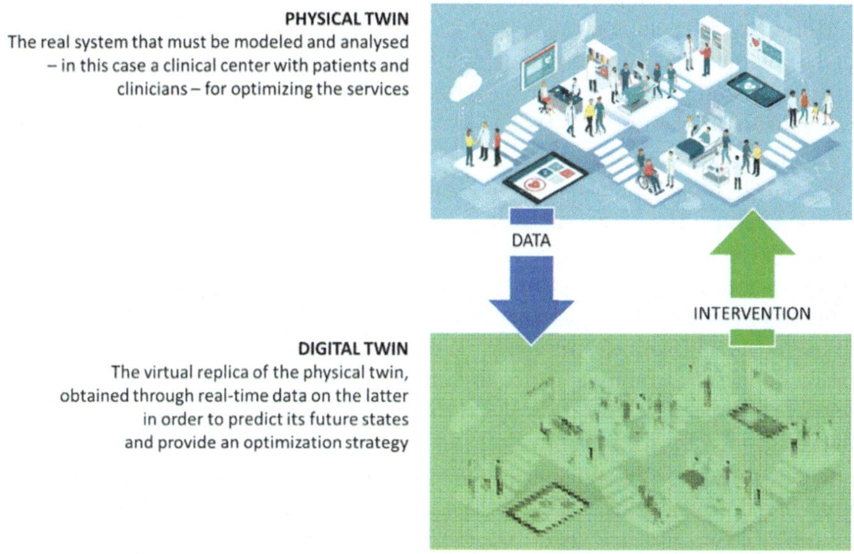


**Fig. 1** This illustration depicts the hypothetical case of a Digital Twin computationally replicating agents (mainly: patients, clinicians) and events within a hospital. Its objective is to help the experts formulate a strategy for optimizing the healthcare services within the Physical Twin

Twin usually exists before someone creates its Digital Twin; the (raw and processed) data are bidirectionally exchanged between the twins and analyzed; each item and its counterpart tend to be synchronized, identical, and physically bound; the Digital Twin can also interface two machines or a human and a machine (human–machine interaction, HMI). Anyway, the ongoing outburst of novel DT-based concepts keeps defying these categories: this is the case of the "Digital Triplet" [29, 30], an AI layer dedicated to assist the human decision-making according to the DT output.

Among the recurring features retrieved in literature, bidirectionality in digital twinning (i.e., the process generating a Digital Twin and its relationship with its physical counterpart) does not constitute an obvious characteristic because a consensus on its definition does not seem concluded. Although many papers refer to "automated bidirectionality," the feedback from Digital Twin to Physical Twin is often based on updating a designer or a manager with information to improve the Physical Twin according to predictions made by playing the Digital Twin during the product life cycle. This is highlighted by observing how a Digital Twin can be defined by its main scope [31]: (i) monitoring the conditions and the features of a Physical Twin, (ii) replicating the future patterns of the Physical Twin states, (iii) establishing direct interactions with a Physical Twin based on a cyber-physical system (in this case, we can talk about "operational Digital Twins"). The latter case could happen, even without any human intervention, through a Physical Twin enriched by actuated components that respond to automatic decisions based on parameters for optimizing the replicated system according to the replica-based predictions [32]. Obviously, such an automated bidirectionality is a feature with high requirements, scaling with the Physical Twin complexity and depending on ubiquitous infrastructures and high-performance telecommunication protocols [31] for managing uncertain conditions in the computationally modeled real settings [33]. Additionally, they need advanced machine learning and deep learning systems to discover or to implement the optimal ways to modify the Physical Twin [34].

Such processes are actively explored in intelligent manufacturing solutions like [35] and, in order to make Digital Twins closer to the real world, [36] in cyber-physical twins. This term emphasizes the environmental influence on the physical object and the feedback from the digital world to the real world. The authors proposed this new type of twins to improve the product development processes, which can be empowered beyond the advantages offered by Digital Twins [37] to make simulated experiments with virtual prototypes. Within this context, an interesting approach is based on the opportunity to program machines through Digital Twins experienced (even in teleoperation conditions) by the expert as the user of intuitive virtual reality interfaces [38]. Such a scenario discloses the potential of these advanced interactive simulations in robotics and human–robot interaction (HRI) [39]. However, there are unexplored ways to make this process more intuitive for the expert [40]. This could become viable by connecting a Digital Twin with a physical replica of the robot constituting part of the Physical Twin (this topic will be treated in the penultimate section of this chapter, within the sub-section on "Phygital Twins") [25]. We can consider this as a result of a trend making physical and virtual items converge [41], especially in case the first are based on an embodied AI like a robot.

Interestingly, the main challenges of Digital Twins in HRI [42] can depend on the difficulty of representing the human component within the human–robot system. Such a barrier becomes even more challenging if we face the complexity of the human health and of the healthcare systems, as next section will discuss.

## 3 Healthcare Applications

The healthcare applications of Digital Twins constitute further challenges for this innovative technology. Indeed, fully modeling human beings (even organs or cells) is certainly beyond the technical capabilities of any device that can be developed nowadays. It is difficult to envision if and when a comprehensive Digital Twin of any living organism can be implemented (especially considering how cognitive-behavioral processes cannot be excluded from the domain of biological systems). However, it is possible to proceed through a pragmatic approach for devising interactive models able to assist the problem-solving procedures in specific subdomains, circumscribing issues that constitute constraints to our actions in understanding and improving the health conditions of a person for implementing precision medicine strategies [11, 43, 44]. Nonetheless, Digital Twins can be exploited in healthcare for modeling not only human beings but also any system, process, and product [45] in order to optimize workflows and to improve clinical performance and health outcomes with minimal risk. Even the experiences of patients, doctors, and other stakeholders can become a target, ameliorating the healthcare services management as well.

Considering these scenarios, next sub-sections will propose exemplary applications of Digital Twins to healthcare, with special attention to the ones of mHealth as framework that remarks the opportunity of collecting data and offering feedback ubiquitously, especially to the patients. These examples constitute preliminary explorations in this field: they offer promising prototypes that can contribute to investigate and improve human health.

### *3.1 Digital Twins for Health*

Figure 2 represents a typical perspective of Digital Twin applications for biomedical research and healthcare: as introduced above, digital human modeling [46] is a real challenge for the current technological constraints. In order to collect information on the patients' conditions and journey, wearable devices and IoT systems provided data should be combined with the ones derived from clinical procedures so as to approach the real-time replication of the individual. The study in [47], focused on the creation of a "perioperative Human Digital Twin," lists different types of data that can be exploited for accomplishing this task:

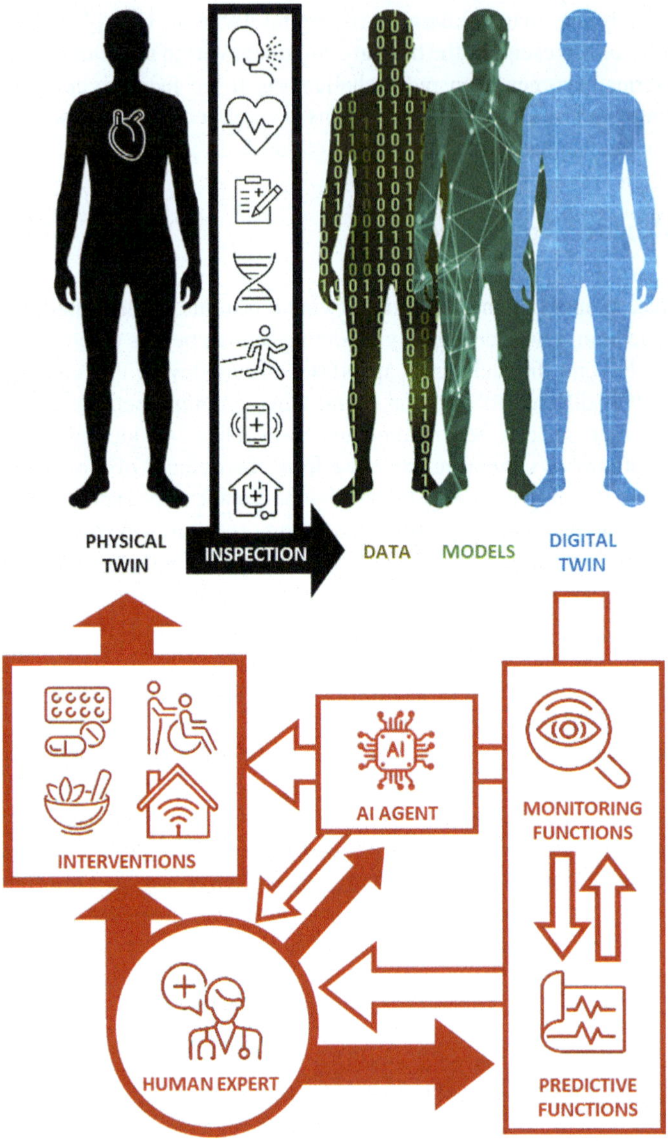


**Fig. 2** A representation of the potential steps in Digital Twin generation and exploitation. The latter can be performed by AI systems and/or a human expert (e.g., clinician, researcher). It is also necessary to make the interventions automatic through digital feedback or mechatronic actuation (technically, these AI systems can be part of the Digital Twin itself within a cyber-physical system). However, human experts should always check the decisions implemented by the AI

- clinical electronic documentation,
- results of laboratory tests (including genotyping) and bioimaging,
- psychological tests (with special attention to stress and mood),
- patient-reported outcomes,
- medication consumption,
- remote patient monitoring,
- data from wearable devices for health tracking,
- exposomic data (from pollution to diet and urban safety),
- social media (e.g., text mining through Natural Language Processing),
- technology use habits (from smartphones to refrigerator),
- GPS (e.g., time spent on the gym and on the ice-cream store).

The authors [47] also discussed a set of requirements for generating Human Digital Twin that could display just information with high relevance for clinical decision-making. These Human Digital Twins should be based on features (partially discussed in terms of ethical issues in the third section of this chapter too) like

- seamless integration into the clinical activities described into the actual workflow (without being unobtrusive and difficult to use);
- being widely available and affordable;
- interoperability between different systems for clinicians and patients;
- large evidence basis for the validation of their output (that should work as digital biomarkers and as recommendations for treatments);
- iterative processing for continuous learning to refine models of individuals and populations during the individual treatments;
- capability to accommodate all available source-independent data;
- reliable automated solutions for dealing with missing information;
- ability to mitigate biases inherently present in clinical data;
- standards of data security and privacy.

Overall, the largest set of individual data (potentially compatible with information from novel sources) we can afford according to the current limitations in information processing should be used for facing challenges like managing a viral infection [48], monitoring and anticipating the life course of an individual [49], predicting the therapeutic outcomes for developing novel pharmacological treatments [50], improving our own methodologies in biomedical research [51]—indeed, Digital Twins can be used by healthcare services and in scientific investigations as well. Another example can be based on the need of predicting the response to treatments during the first 24 h of sepsis [52] through the advanced computational implementation of mathematical models and algorithms for replicating events across multiple functional stages of major systems in the human body (cardiovascular system, neurologic system, renal system, respiratory system, gastrointestinal system, blood system) and their inflammatory responses. Relevant biomarkers are visualized for enabling the medical doctors to take decisions on next interventions according to the patient's expected responses, predicted according to the Digital Twins output.

Any Digital Twin of patients and their biological systems (from a cell to the person as a whole) can be exploited in different ways. Achieving a Digital Patient [53] is a strategy explored in multiple medical domains. It can focus on the heterogeneous effects and issues of a specific disease, as in the cases discussed by Voigt et al. [54], on Multiple Sclerosis, demonstrating the multiple types of data that Digital Twins can be applied in this domain in various ways. For instance, they can work as individualized innovative disease management solutions for helping people with multiple sclerosis to cope with the quite unpredictable progression of this disease, hitting different sensory, cognitive, and motor functions. AI techniques for the analysis of disease parameters—e.g., medical procedures, clinical and para-clinical outcomes, biomarkers, patient-related data, information on the individual life circumstances and plans, multi-omics—can generate a Digital Twin that can be coupled with the patient's characteristics. Such a virtual replica can help the clinicians to handle large and complex datasets as coherent predictive information on degenerative diseases, contributing to a personalized healthcare plan. Such an approach may lead to standardized procedures for achieving individual clinical pathways, even supporting the clinician-patient communication to facilitate a shared decision-making process.

Digital Patients can also be adopted for appropriately improve highly critical procedures like surgeries [55, 56]. In such a domain, the Digital Twin of a patient can be used for helping a physician or a team of doctors during activities like planning an operation or getting practice about a procedure on a specific individual (beyond the effectiveness of any simulator for the training of medical residents). The review in [57] discussed, for instance, the potential role of Digital Twins in improving the procedures for arthroscopic surgery education through the integration of diagnostic data, bioimaging, surgical practice, and intraoperative data. This would enable surgical skills training, preoperative planning, and novel databases of surgical simulations. The predictive capabilities of Digital Twins can also be employed for anticipating the consequences of surgeries. For example, the authors of [58] considered post-hepatectomy portal hypertension as a major cause of liver failure leading to death. This defines the need of accurately predicting such a complication for each patient. Thus, they proposed and tested (on a cohort of 47 patients undergoing major hepatectomy) a mathematical model implemented as a Digital Twin-like solution predicting the portocaval gradient at the end of the liver resection. The authors demonstrated that their Digital Twin prototype can inform the physicians for modifying the currently adopted algorithms for surgical decision-making.

Considering general medical decision-making, [59] discusses another aspect of the potential applications of Digital Twins in health domains: improving the workflow efficiency in a large medical procedural suite of Electronic Health Record systems. In such contexts, many processes could become erroneous, impairing the individual capability (and increasing the frustration of the medical doctors) to manage and optimize the workflow in real time. The authors proposed a Digital Twin of the procedural suite enabling the process of making data-driven decisions, providing gastroenterology outpatient centers with long-term improvements.

Another example of medical optimization can be based on approaching the domains of Health Technology Assessment (HTA) and medical devices usability engineering. Indeed, Digital Twins could also be advantageous for virtually representing and assessing a medical device before planning and performing its clinical trials. This strategy could work for mitigating any predictable risk before the trials themselves. In [60], the authors address and discuss this, specifically referring to the development of endoscopic medical devices for minimally invasive screening and intervention. After facing ethical and safety considerations about in vivo animal studies and clinical trials for the evaluation of these systems, the authors propose the computational digital modeling of biological tissues and processes, medical devices, and their interactions in order to provide a set of cost-effective solutions for accelerating the evaluation of endoscopic devices and minimizing most risks in these procedures.

According to their observations, the development of a Digital Twin including the human gastrointestinal tract requires the reconstruction of the complex intestinal geometry according to medical images and a multi-physics model replicating the in vivo systems and processes. Certainly, the complexity in these items represents the most current criticalities in the adoption of Digital Twin in healthcare, and they can be extended to the medical device personalization.

These examples certainly play a role within the organization of a healthcare center like a hospital. The complexity of these contexts additionally increases the burden of any Digital Twin that could be proposed for anticipating and managing the potential issues in a place inhabited by patients in heterogeneous conditions at different degrees of severity and by professionals operating on these critical situations. However, the impact of Digital Twin can surely be disruptive in improving the care processes, as in the trauma management cases discussed in [61] for introducing the opportunity to use intelligent agents in healthcare. The authors proposed innovation solutions for Digital Twins, integrating frameworks and approaches for modeling and design with computational agents.

They also foresaw a roadmap of research in this domain: investigating semantic models supporting agent reasoning about Digital Twins; pondering how agent-based Digital Twins could be helpful for devising and improving the future healthcare information architecture systems and standards; defining simulations to support the agent's decision-making. This certainly includes even the information retrieval and the data mining for the Decision Support System (DSS) in medical domains [62].

Thus, Digital Twins can optimize processes at different scales (e.g., replicating cybersecurity criticalities) [63], encompassing smart environments (from the Hospital 4.0 to a Smart City) as in IoMT settings [64] (including homes enriched by sensors and systems for ambient intelligence). They can even simulate apparently narrow problems like the pathways of patients [65] or surely widespread ones like the safety of elder people [66, 67]. Even the vaccination centers during the COVID-19 pandemic emergency were analyzed to be represented by Digital Twins [68]. The reference to the pandemic is not casual: the stress experienced by the healthcare systems forced the scientific-technological community to propose novel ways for optimizing the allocation of resources among frail people at risk.

This situation pushed the need of presenting solutions of sustainable and resilient healthcare based on decentralized services supported by approaches like

Telemedicine (including robotic systems for remote rehabilitation), Digital Health, and services of Connected Care, especially for older adults [69–72]. This situation unveiled the need of considering the complexity of these phenomena within wider frameworks like the One Digital Health to shape future technological ecosystems [73], starting with Smart Cities designed (and modeled through Digital Twins) for sustaining health and well-being through cost-effective solutions for countering public emergencies too [74].

Interestingly, these solutions do not necessarily require advanced and expensive systems. Even if major research efforts should be made to propose effective Digital Twins for health in terms of capability to perform real-time simulations, even the currently common device like a smartphone can become a medium for exploiting their potential.

Next sub-section will discuss this point, showing how mHealth can be an exemplary domain of application of Digital Twin technologies, especially considering the patients' journey.

### *3.2 An Exemplary Domain: mHealth*

About mHealth, it is obviously possible to consider the mobile devices (and many wearable devices) as one of the classes of information sources that may update a Digital Twin, monitoring the conditions of a patient (in order to inform the latter or a clinician) or of a wider system (e.g., home, hospital, city). For example, the study in [75] proposed a Digital Twin prototype for analyzing the requirements (low latency, high reliability, high security levels) of telecommunication in a critical application of remote surgery supported by mobile networks.

Digital Twins can also work for providing the Physical Twin with feedback aiming at intervening for a positive change. However, there are peculiarities in Digital Twin for mHealth that derive from the capability of mobile systems to be personal and portable, following "everyone everywhere." For instance, the research in [76] aimed at exploring the perceptions of a 3D Digital Twin representing the anatomy of a person through a mobile application designed for promoting a behavior change in terms of health and weight management. Thus, this type of mHealth apps can exploit Digital Twin technologies through the advantages of mobile systems—convenience, easy access, automatic progress monitoring for delivering solutions addressing issues of societal concern like the obesity increase. Literature has already remarked how avatars based on digital replicas—as the Digital Twins can be—of individuals can engage people in thinking about themselves and their difficulties, from emotion regulation to weight management. These virtual representations, experienced through mobile devices too [77–82], can be helpful for persuading the users in changing their behaviors in several contexts of daily life (thanks to the device portability). The authors in [76] moved their investigations from such a background to remark the importance of detailed and realistic depictions of one's body as one of the main guidelines in this type of applications of Digital Twins. Indeed, they propose to focus upcoming research on the individual differences in anthropomorphism perception [83], a suggestion that can lead to advances in personalization and adaptive features of Digital Twins supported by mHealth apps for the patients. Extensive follow-up studies with large sample size would be necessary, anyway, for clarifying the impact of these solutions, possibly disclosing the opportunity to release further applications of these approaches for mitigating the effects of chronic diseases, improving the individual self-care attitude by providing the users with visual information on their current conditions and their potential change over time. Such a scenario could mitigate health risks through a persuasive and pervasive use of these technologies.

These applications probably tend to elicit the same processes underlying the effects of game-based solutions for health [84], based, for instance, on making the person aware of the consequences of their actions (feeling competent and "in charge") and, possibly, sharing these information with other individuals. Obviously, proposing any gamification (adopting engaging game-like features in applications that are designed for scopes not including the leisure—e.g., exercise and education) feature could be premature without an adequate series of studies. It is not strange that this is envisioned even in applications using virtual reality settings and Digital Twins for construction safety training [85].

However, they could become one of the many components of a multi-faceted technological ecosystem for health [86] where each patient can experience the feeling of being involved in the care processes by making them aware of their conditions and of their options in decision-making through portable, personal, engaging solutions [47]. Such a scenario could exploit the data collected on a person to generate multiple Digital Twins, designed in specific ways for the well-being and the scopes of the user (patient, for self-care, or physician, for diagnostics), interconnecting them where it would be appropriate and useful.

Beyond these applications targeting individual users (even if groups engaging tasks through the same mHealth app including Digital Twins of each member can be envisioned), Digital Twins can be developed [87] for assisting the strategies of decentralization in healthcare systems (a remedy to their overload), especially exploiting wider networks including mobile systems, wearables, IoMT, and smart environments. This approach would lead to an improvement of the healthcare system sustainability by spreading virtual replicas of the patients and of any person at risk (and everyone is at health risk even through a healthy aging process) who can find easy and acceptable the usage of a smartphone. However, the usability and the acceptance of Digital Twins can raise further issues that are introduced in next section.

## 4 Human-Centric Perspectives

The panorama of Digital Twin solutions for healthcare is certainly rich of different options for helping patients, clinicians, researchers, and anyone involved in this domain for ameliorating the health conditions of individuals and groups. Obviously, improvements can be made. Aside from the technical enhancements of sensors capabilities, computational power, connection reliability, and speed, there are aspects that must be addressed in order to be ready for the introduction of these technologies. Handling these issues requires a "human-centric" perspective that must lead any healthcare 4.0 system to appropriately serve its users [88, 89]. In this domain, such a point of view is intrinsically based on approaches promoting the engagement of patients and stakeholders (especially in terms of collaboration), the growth in awareness of one's health, the competitive advantage of systems like hospitals in terms of care and costs. Accordingly, a methodological and paradigmatic shift toward the centrality of the person can be helpful to envision how to improve the Digital Twin systems even before their most recent technical features will be implemented (possibly predicting the problems that could be generated by them). Next sections will present two examples of human-centric topics in this discussion.

The first one will focus on a potential strategy to improve the experience of the experts interacting with a Digital Twin by adding "phygital" features to it. The focus on Digital Twin users (e.g., clinicians, researchers) is quite advantageous for involving them in the decision-making processes, considering the complexity of handling a virtual system that can affect the real one. The proposed solution can be seen as an insight offered to "twinning designers" that could be inspired to further exploit the convergent technologies supporting the Digital Twins for easing the interaction of the experts with the virtual models of health-related systems.

The second one will be dedicated to the ethical issues raised by Digital Twins as "tentative" replicas of human beings or of systems bringing sensitive data on individuals and groups. These issues must be managed far before the introduction of novel technologies into the market and in any real use context. Such a perspective is definitely human-centric: it pays attention to problems that could be generated by the introduction of novel technologies, enabling actions and situations that could not have been expected by the developers or by any stakeholders.

## *4.1 Beyond Digital Twins: Phygital Twins*

A recent opinion paper proposed the term "Phygital Twins" in neuroergonomics (the discipline that, according to neuroscientific methods, investigates and improves the interactions between a person and the other elements of a system) applied to HRI design [25]. This neologism—previously used in [90] to label an IoT setup collecting data to depict an environment in precision agriculture applications—refers to the opportunity of blending physical and real dimensions in "phygital" spaces and interactions [91, 92], possibly as extensions of Tactile User Interfaces (TUIs) within a general trend of virtuality-reality confluence [41] that involves healthcare too [93]. Interestingly, such a trend matches the expectations underlying the most recent ways to define the metaverse, a digital world possibly encompassing and intertwining cyber-physical systems and Digital Twins with their connection with the real world [94].

In operative terms, Fig. 3 depicts an example of Phygital Twin based on [25]. In this case, the Physical Twin is based on a system including an exoskeleton and its user. Such a system can be fully replicated by a Digital Twin that does not enable any physical interaction or by a Phygital Twin, which replicates just certain components of its real counterpart as digital objects. The other components are replicated by physical objects. Overall, the digital and physical replicas are integrated within an extended reality model. In this model, the physical objects are constituted by instances of the same product (it could be any kind of physical system, certainly not only robots) in the Physical Twin. Both digital and phygital settings are experienced by a remote expert through a headset for mixed reality. In this example, such a setup enables a live visualization of anomalies in the right shoulder muscles of the wearable robot user.

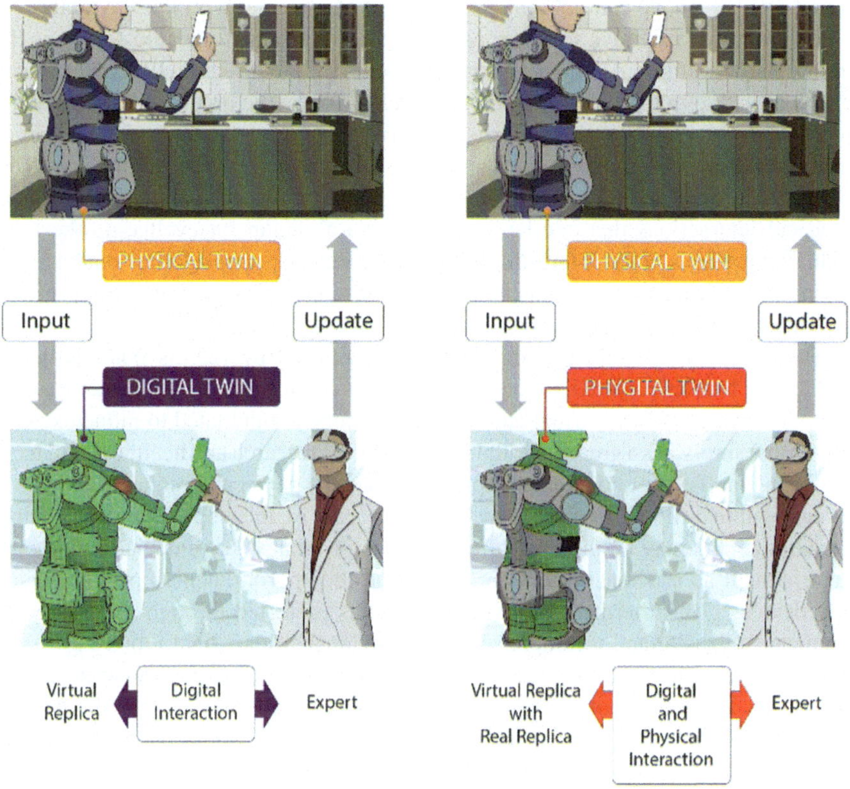


**Fig. 3** On the top of the image—adapted from [25] we show a human-exoskeleton system within a use context. This Physical Twin is connected to the bottom twins. Left: a Digital Twin (in green)—this is a virtual replica of the system on top. Right: a Phygital Twin—a "holographic" replica of the device user on a mannequin "wearing" a second exoskeleton into a laboratory. The smartphone held by the user is employed to collect data and to interact with the exoskeleton and with the remote expert assessing the situation for improving the device settings

Differently from the case of the Digital Twin, the expert interacting with the Phygital Twin can influence the model and test its future states through intuitive physical interactions with haptic feedback offered by a real exoskeleton. Importantly, the case presented in Fig. 3 shows the exoskeleton user interacting with a mobile phone, enabling (beyond any data collection of their conditions) a communication with the remote expert. Through this channel, the exoskeleton user can provide or negate the informed consent to receive any update of the wearable robot software based on the Phygital Twin predictions and the expert decisions.

Overall, the physical components of the Phygital Twin would facilitate the assessment and the management of the Physical Twin, and they would replicate their counterparts with higher reliability than any digital model because they are constituted by the same items. Further computer-generated objects and settings may also be integrated in the visual scene in a virtual environment fully surrounding the user. Furthermore, another phone can help the remote expert to interact with the Phygital Twin without a fully immersive scenario, especially for focusing on specific details on the individual conditions. About the latter, the paper in [25] focused on HRI contexts with exemplary cases akin to Phygital Twins in fields like bionic prosthetics [95, 96] and rehabilitation technologies [97], envisioning the generation of quantifiable indices of healthy and pathological conditions or response to treatments: digital biomarkers [98] becoming a "phygital biomarker" thanks to the informational components based on physical interactions that can be exploited by a clinician for evaluating the individual conditions [69]. Interestingly, novel frameworks considering dual Digital Twins representing patients and clinicians within a tele-rehabilitation setting already provide scenarios that can take advantage of this approach [72].

However, the "twinning design" concept proposed by [25] is potentially not limited to human-centered robot design and evaluation into a "meta-laboratory" (a hybrid context where virtual and real items can be manipulated to influence each other) that surely has a great potential for biomedical research and healthcare. Indeed, any item that (before and after its deployment) can be physically replicated and integrated within a Phygital Twin may constitute part of the implementation of this paradigm. This may be the case of an assistive or rehabilitative device, or a home environment as a whole, especially for testing the appropriateness of introducing IoT devices [70] in terms of individual reactions (detected through data collected by means of distal and wearable sensors). Obviously, this would require a certain level of actuation in the Physical Twin, but this could become an important option for easing the activity of a remote clinician or researcher desiring to modify the surroundings of a frail person in order to evaluate their conditions or for anticipating the interventions to be adopted when certain symptoms initiate to occur [69]. Certainly, this approach can be used for evaluating medical devices too, especially (as in the example) robotic systems. It would also be interesting to predict the learning performance of health tech users and clinical trainees, but it is important to not let the enthusiasm for modeling exceed in computationally depicting and, hazardously, de-personalizing any human being. Such a situation would be detrimental in terms of human-centric design: involving people and considering holistically their setting would not be enough to counter any fall in catching the value of the person represented by a software-based model. This last point leads to the next sub-section, dedicated to ethical issues in twinning processes and their results.

## 4.2 *Ethical Issues in Twinning for Health*

The technologies supporting these paradigms surely have limitations: replicating live processes in ecologically valid contexts surely brings a computational burden, preceded by the connectivity issues generated by the effort of approaching real-time conditions. However, Digital Twins also raise a series of questions that must be faced for introducing them in real contexts, pondering topics like technology acceptance [99]. Ethical issues are certainly among the problems that should be considered before planning the development of any technological solution in order to make it truly human-centric, especially when we consider situations requiring quick decision-making processes as in several healthcare procedures [61] and, in general, most precision medicine scenarios that are considered by HTA [100].

Accordingly, the authors of [101] proposed an "ethical map" of the potential ethical issues that Digital Twin could generate. According to this map, there could be sources of ethical issues in data collection (data quality, and unorthodox use of data), data management (ownership and accessibility of data, brokerage, hacking), data analysis (biased algorithms, biased training data set), information use (disease decontextualization, epistemic injustice, over-diagnosis). These items can lead to heterogeneous issues, encompassing the distortion of the physician's diagnosis or the distortion of the patient's body image, and even detrimental effects on the doctor-patient relationship. Further issues can affect the privacy and the consent in data authoring, representation, storage, and use: the standardization of these aspects should aim at assuring that only authorized people can access and edit personal information on patients. Even the definitions of concepts like normality, enhancement, and extension of human beings must be pondered. These themes cross domains encompassing engineering and philosophy [102].

For instance, [103] discusses how the requests for personalized medicine of fine grained information on individuals can be supported by the exploitation of Digital Twins to assess the emerging data-driven healthcare practices, even pondering their implications for therapy, preventive care, and human augmentation. However, representing the physiological state and the habits of a person over time leads to the need of reflecting on what we consider a therapeutic intervention or an enhancement procedure: while these technologies emerge, we must carefully define the risks on these aspects, pointing at the concept of normality (difficultly depicted through quantitative parameters in most cases). Thinking about these issues is a premise to weight the societal impact of Digital Twins alongside other criticalities as in the domains of transparency and privacy in data usage.

On the other hand, [104] highlights the concrete challenges posed by Digital Twins in terms of interactions between people and their virtual counterparts before discussing how a digital item may replicate a person. The author interestingly analyzes the peculiarities of Digital Twins, remarking their dynamic quality in co-adapting with their Physical Twins. The focus on human beings, especially about their health and value, is particularly demonstrated by the attention in depicting the relationships between physical and simulated worlds as bidirectional activities: representation and control. This is especially important for clarifying how the Digital Twins can be depicted as a way to influence the people and the organizations they model through their predictive power, generating potential concerns (in particular considering the possibility of having an embodied replica that could be perceived as an extension of the original body). The author discusses how Digital Twins do not fundamentally threaten the individual integrity, and their challenges are affordable. However, it could be critically important to consider the opportunity for a person to have control over their simulated representation. This implies the need of a dynamic consent (mimicking the dynamic quality of twinning itself), enabling a person to approve to be represented by a Digital Twin, even selecting if this is allowed for therapy or for health prediction. However, if a person does not have control over their Digital Twin (or they are not aware of it), this could become an illegitimate representation, approaching the perception of a shift toward an inappropriate surveillance. Even if this latter aspect can be countered by solutions of privacy-by-design and value-sensitive design typically discussed in contexts of IoT and ambient intelligence [70] and in the ubiquitous and pervasive scenarios of IoMT and mHealth [105], it is definitely important to consider their potential impact to define a responsible way to deal with any emergent technology enabling novel paradigms of modeling and interaction. Interestingly, the proposal in [104] to employ embodied machines for enabling the person to have a true interaction with their computational model matches the user-centered proposal of the aforementioned Phygital Twins of the previous subsection: this way, a solution proposed for easing an expert (e.g., clinician, researcher, designer, manager) in the fruition of a technological representation can help solving a morally sensitive issue for a patient. These are among the conditions that, according to the author, can make a Digital Twin an ethically justifiable form of human (and human health) representation. It would be wise to discuss them within the dialectics about the factors facilitating or restraining the adoption of twinning procedures [106].

As suggested above, the human-centric role of these issues is based on the opportunity to anticipate potential problems (possibly through design guidelines and standardization policies) for the human capabilities and dignity while even pondering the opportunities offered by innovations that never cease to create innovative frameworks from the confluence of different technologies [107].

## 5 Conclusion

The advantages of emulating and simulating complex systems are certainly obvious: it is possible to investigate a digital model representing a complex system by imitating its behavior and its inner structure. The most recent data-intensive network-based computing solutions are enabling a further revolution through the Digital Twins: real-time replicas of physical systems that can be analyzed in their current and future states in order to influence them (according to the decisions of humans or intelligent agents or, synergistically, both). Digital Twins definitely represent a revolution in exploring the potential confluence of a variety of solutions for data collection and analysis, computational modeling, and interaction design for practical scopes. Surely, they can ease our way to handle complexities from the scale of tissues to one of cities. Obviously, the promises of Digital Twins need further investigations, especially pondering their human-centric aspects.

This is especially true when we consider the applications of Digital Twins in healthcare domains—for instance: understanding the potential paths of a disease progression in individuals for adapting a therapy or for evaluating and optimizing the allocation of resources across a community during a pandemic particularly hitting the elderly population, assessing and improving the control of robotic medical devices according to the data collected from users with disabilities. Replicating organs, individuals, medical devices, or even a hospital can be successful examples of a strategy that needs novel sources of data and channel of intervention for refining its contribution to the frameworks enabling precision medicine and connected care.

In particular, mHealth offers unique opportunities for developing Digital Twins of mobile users and of the systems within they act. This approach aims at predicting and managing the system conditions through personal data and interventions that can be, respectively, gathered and provided ubiquitously, literally following the person and interacting with the surrounding devices. In particular, it discusses the personal use of an implementation of a Digital Twin as the avatar of a mobile user, specifically a patient who can find the visualization of the simulacrum as a solution to elicit attitude and proactivity for self-care.

This chapter presented introductory perspectives on this kind of scenario as an overview of opportunities and critical aspects that must be handled to fully benefit from these novel technological solutions even before their actual development and access to the market. Easing the work of clinical experts in interacting with an intuitive Phygital Twin and facing the ethical issues intrinsically tied to the twinning process and its results are just two examples of human-centric aspects that must be pondered in this domain. Through these exemplary (critical and purposeful) perspectives, Digital Twins can also work as an interface with our well-being, the medical devices, and the healthcare services.

## References


1. McGregor, I.: The relationship between simulation and emulation. In: Proceedings of the Winter Simulation Conference, IEEE, pp 1683–1688 (2002)
2. Hsu, Y., Chiu, J.-M., Liu, J.S.: Digital twins for industry 4.0 and beyond. In: 2019 IEEE International Conference on Industrial Engineering and Engineering Management (IEEM), IEEE, pp 526–530 (2019)

3. Bagaria, N., Laamarti, F., Badawi, H.F., Albraikan, A., Martinez Velazquez, R.A., El Saddik, A.: Health 4.0: digital twins for health and well-being. In: Connected Health in Smart Cities, pp. 143–152. Springer (2020)
4. Phanden, R.K., Sharma, P., Dubey, A.: A review on simulation in digital twin for aerospace, manufacturing and robotics. Mater. Today: Proc. **38**, 174–178 (2021)
5. Juarez, M.G., Botti, V.J., Giret, A.S.: Digital twins: review and challenges. J. Comput. Inf. Sci. Eng. 21(3) (2021)
6. Ritto, T., Rochinha, F.: Digital twin, physics-based model, and machine learning applied to damage detection in structures. Mech. Syst. Signal Process. **155**, 107614 (2021)
7. Allam, Z., Bibri, S.E., Jones, D.S., Chabaud, D., Moreno, C.: Unpacking the '15-Minute City'via 6G, IoT, and digital twins: towards a new narrative for increasing urban efficiency, resilience, and sustainability. Sensors **22**(4), 1369 (2022)
8. Jiang, J., Tobia, M., Lawther, R., Branchaud, D., Bednarz, T.: Double vision: digital twin applications within extended reality. In: ACM SIGGRAPH 2020 Appy Hour, pp. 1–2 (2020)
9. Coorey, G., Figtree, G.A., Fletcher, D.F., Redfern, J.: The health digital twin: advancing precision cardiovascular medicine. Nat. Rev. Cardiol. **18**(12), 803–804 (2021)
10. Li, X., Liu, H., Wang, W., Zheng, Y., Lv, H., Lv, Z.: Big data analysis of the internet of things in the digital twins of smart city based on deep learning. Futur. Gener. Comput. Syst. **128**, 167–177 (2022)
11. Ahmadi-Assalemi, G., Al-Khateeb, H., Maple, C., Epiphaniou, G., Alhaboby, Z.A., Alkaabi, S., Alhaboby, D.: Digital twins for precision healthcare. In: Cyber Defence in the Age of AI, Smart Societies and Augmented Humanity. Springer, pp 133–158 (2020)
12. Evjemo, L.D., Gjerstad, T., Grøtli, E.I., Sziebig, G.: Trends in smart manufacturing: role of humans and industrial robots in smart factories. Curr. Robot. Rep. **1**(2), 35–41 (2020)
13. Yang, D., Karimi, H.R., Kaynak, O., Yin, S.: Developments of digital twin technologies in industrial, smart city and healthcare sectors: a survey. Complex Eng. Syst. **1**(1), 3 (2021)
14. Guo, J., Lv, Z.: Application of digital twins in multiple fields. Multim. Tools Appl. 1–27 (2022)
15. Qiu, C., Zhou, S., Liu, Z., Gao, Q., Tan, J.: Digital assembly technology based on augmented reality and digital twins: a review. Virtual Real. Intell. Hardw. **1**(6), 597–610 (2019)
16. Jeršov, S., Tepljakov, A.: Digital twins in extended reality for control system applications. In: 2020 43rd International Conference on Telecommunications and Signal Processing (TSP). IEEE, pp 274–279 (2020)
17. Madhavan, S., Beckman, R.A., McCoy, M.D., Pishvaian, M.J., Brody, J.R., Macklin, P.: Envisioning the future of precision oncology trials. Nat. Cancer **2**(1), 9–11 (2021)
18. Grieves, M., Vickers, J.: Digital twin: mitigating unpredictable, undesirable emergent behavior in complex systems. In: Transdisciplinary perspectives on complex systems. Springer, pp. 85–113 (2017)
19. Shafto, M., Conroy, M., Doyle, R., Glaessgen, E., Kemp, C., LeMoigne, J., Wang, L.: Modeling, simulation, information technology & processing roadmap. Natl. Aeronaut. Space Adm. **32**(2012), 1–38 (2012)
20. Jones, D., Snider, C., Nassehi, A., Yon, J., Hicks, B.: Characterising the digital twin: a systematic literature review. CIRP J. Manuf. Sci. Technol. **29**, 36–52 (2020)
21. Singh, M., Fuenmayor, E., Hinchy, E.P., Qiao, Y., Murray, N., Devine, D.: Digital twin: origin to future. Appl. Syst. Innov. **4**(2), 36 (2021)
22. Kuehner, K.J., Scheer, R., Strassburger, S.: Digital twin: finding common ground—A meta-review. Procedia CIRP **104**, 1227–1232 (2021)
23. Rossmann, A., Hertweck, D.: Digital twins: a meta-review on their conceptualization, application, and reference architecture
24. Fuller, A., Fan, Z., Day, C., Barlow, C.: Digital twin: enabling technologies, challenges and open research. IEEE Access **8**, 108952–108971 (2020)
25. Barresi, G., Pacchierotti, C., Laffranchi, M., De Michieli, L.: Beyond digital twins: phygital twins for neuroergonomics in human-robot interaction. Front. Neurorobot. 138 (2022)

26. Kritzinger, W., Karner, M., Traar, G., Henjes, J., Sihn, W.: Digital twin in manufacturing: a categorical literature review and classification. IFAC-PapersOnLine **51**(11), 1016–1022 (2018)
27. Semeraro, C., Lezoche, M., Panetto, H., Dassisti, M.: Digital twin paradigm: a systematic literature review. Comput. Ind. **130**, 103469 (2021)
28. Van der Valk, H., Haße, H., Möller, F., Arbter, M., Henning, J.-L., Otto, B.: A taxonomy of digital Twins. In: AMCIS (2020)
29. Gichane, M.M., Byiringiro, J.B., Chesang, A.K., Nyaga, P.M., Langat, R.K., Smajic, H., Kiiru, C.W.: Digital triplet approach for real-time monitoring and control of an elevator security system. Designs **4**(2), 9 (2020)
30. Umeda, Y., Ota, J., Kojima, F., Saito, M., Matsuzawa, H., Sukekawa, T., Takeuchi, A., Makida, K., Shirafuji, S.: Development of an education program for digital manufacturing system engineers based on 'Digital Triplet'concept. Procedia Manuf. **31**, 363–369 (2019)
31. Khan, L.U., Saad, W., Niyato, D., Han, Z., Hong, C.S.: Digital-twin-enabled 6G: vision, architectural trends, and future directions. IEEE Commun. Mag. **60**(1), 74–80 (2022)
32. Liu, Y., Ong, S, Nee, A.: State-of-the-art survey on digital twin implementations. Adv. Manuf. 1–23 (2022)
33. Barricelli, B.R., Casiraghi, E., Fogli, D.: A survey on digital twin: definitions, characteristics, applications, and design implications. IEEE Access **7**, 167653–167671 (2019)
34. Groshev, M., Guimarães, C., Martín-Pérez, J., de la Oliva, A.: Toward intelligent cyber-physical systems: digital twin meets artificial intelligence. IEEE Commun. Mag. **59**(8), 14–20 (2021)
35. Wang, T., Li, J., Deng, Y., Wang, C., Snoussi, H., Tao, F.: Digital twin for human-machine interaction with convolutional neural network. Int. J. Comput. Integr. Manuf. **34**(7–8), 888–897 (2021)
36. Czwick, C., Anderl, R.: Cyber-physical twins-definition, conception and benefit. Procedia CIRP **90**, 584–588 (2020)
37. Haag, S., Anderl, R.: Digital twin–Proof of concept. Manuf. Lett. **15**, 64–66 (2018)
38. Burghardt, A., Szybicki, D., Gierlak, P., Kurc, K., Pietruś, P., Cygan, R.: Programming of industrial robots using virtual reality and digital twins. Appl. Sci. **10**(2), 486 (2020)
39. Pairet, È., Ardón, P., Liu, X., Lopes, J., Hastie, H., Lohan, K.S.: A digital twin for human-robot interaction. In: 2019 14th ACM/IEEE International Conference on Human-Robot Interaction (HRI). IEEE, pp 372–372 (2019)
40. Ravichandar, H., Polydoros, A.S., Chernova, S., Billard, A.: Recent advances in robot learning from demonstration. Ann. Rev. Contr., Robot. Auton. Syst. **3**, 297–330 (2020)
41. Tao, F., Zhang, M.: Digital twin shop-floor: a new shop-floor paradigm towards smart manufacturing. IEEE Access **5**, 20418–20427 (2017)
42. Malik, A.A., Bilberg, A.: Digital twins of human robot collaboration in a production setting. Procedia Manuf. **17**, 278–285 (2018)
43. Fagherazzi, G.: Deep digital phenotyping and digital twins for precision health: time to dig deeper. J. Med. Internet Res. **22**(3), e16770 (2020)
44. Booyse, W., Wilke, D.N., Heyns, S.: Deep digital twins for detection, diagnostics and prognostics. Mech. Syst. Signal Process. **140**, 106612 (2020)
45. Elkefi, S., Asan, O.: Digital twins for managing health care systems: rapid literature review. J. Med. Internet Res. **24**(8), e37641 (2022)
46. Paul, G., Abele, N.D., Kluth, K.: A review and qualitative meta-analysis of digital human modeling and cyber-physical-systems in ergonomics 4.0. IISE Trans. Occup. Ergon. Human Factors 1–13 (2021)
47. Lonsdale, H., Gray, G.M., Ahumada, L.M., Yates, H.M., Varughese, A., Rehman, M.A.: The perioperative human digital twin. Anesth. Analg. **134**(4), 885–892 (2022)
48. Laubenbacher, R., Sluka, J.P., Glazier, J.A.: Using digital twins in viral infection. Science **371**(6534), 1105–1106 (2021)
49. Milne-Ives, M., Fraser, L.K., Khan, A., Walker, D., van Velthoven, M.H., May, J., Wolfe, I., Harding, T., Meinert, E.: Life course digital twins-intelligent monitoring for early and

continuous intervention and prevention (LifeTIME): proposal for a retrospective cohort study. JMIR Res. Protoc. **11**(5), e35738 (2022)
50. Subramanian, K.: Digital twin for drug discovery and development—The virtual liver. J. Indian Inst. Sci. **100**(4), 653–662 (2020)
51. Schwartz, S.M., Wildenhaus, K., Bucher, A., Byrd, B.: Digital twins and the emerging science of self: Implications for digital health experience design and "small" data. Front. Comput. Sci. **2**, 31 (2020)
52. Lal, A., Li, G., Cubro, E., Chalmers, S., Li, H., Herasevich, V., Dong, Y., Pickering, B.W., Kilickaya, O., Gajic, O.: Development and verification of a digital twin patient model to predict specific treatment response during the first 24 hours of sepsis. Crit. Care Explor. **2**(11) (2020)
53. Erol, T., Mendi, A.F., Doğan, D.: The digital twin revolution in healthcare. In: 2020 4th International Symposium on Multidisciplinary Studies and Innovative Technologies (ISMSIT), IEEE, pp. 1–7 (2020)
54. Voigt, I., Inojosa, H., Dillenseger, A., Haase, R., Akgün, K., Ziemssen, T.: Digital twins for multiple sclerosis. Front. Immunol. **12**, 1556 (2021)
55. Ahmed, H., Devoto, L.: The potential of a digital twin in surgery. Surg. Innov. **28**(4), 509–510 (2021)
56. Tai, Y., Zhang, L., Li, Q., Zhu, C., Chang, V., Rodrigues, J.J., Guizani, M.: Digital twin-enabled IoMT system for surgical simulation using rAC-GAN. IEEE Internet Things J. (2022)
57. Bjelland, Ø., Rasheed, B., Schaathun, H.G., Pedersen, M.D., Steinert, M., Hellevik, A.I., Bye, R.T.: Towards a digital twin for arthroscopic knee surgery: a systematic review. IEEE Access (2022)
58. Golse, N., Joly, F., Combari, P., Lewin, M., Nicolas, Q., Audebert, C., Samuel, D., Allard, M.-A., Cunha, A.S., Castaing, D.: Predicting the risk of post-hepatectomy portal hypertension using a digital twin: a clinical proof of concept. J. Hepatol. **74**(3), 661–669 (2021)
59. Garbey, M., Joerger, G., Furr, S.: Application of digital twin and heuristic computer reasoning to workflow management: gastroenterology outpatient centers study (2022). medRxiv
60. Kalozoumis, P.G., Marino, M., Carniel, E.L., Lakovidis, D.K.: Towards the development of a digital twin for endoscopic medical device testing. In: Digital Twins for Digital Transformation: Innovation in Industry, pp. 113–145. Springer (2022)
61. Croatti, A., Gabellini, M., Montagna, S., Ricci, A.: On the integration of agents and digital twins in healthcare. J. Med. Syst. **44**(9), 1–8 (2020)
62. Patrone, C., Galli, G., Revetria, R.: A state of the art of digital twin and simulation supported by data mining in the healthcare sector. In: Advancing Technology Industrialization Through Intelligent Software Methodologies, Tools and Techniques, pp. 605–615 (2019)
63. Faleiro, R., Pan, L., Pokhrel, S.R., Doss, R.: Digital twin for cybersecurity: towards enhancing cyber resilience. In: International Conference on Broadband Communications, Networks and Systems, pp. 57–76. Springer (2021)
64. Cicirelli, F., Guerrieri, A., Mastroianni, C., Vinci, A.: Emerging internet of things solutions and technologies. Electronics **10**, 1928 (2021). Note: MDPI stays neutral with regard to jurisdictional claims in published
65. Karakra, A., Fontanili, F., Lamine, E., Lamothe, J.: HospiT'Win: a predictive simulation-based digital twin for patients pathways in hospital. In: 2019 IEEE EMBS International Conference on Biomedical & Health Informatics (BHI), IEEE, pp. 1–4 (2019)
66. Zhao, Z., Shen, L., Yang, C., Wu, W., Zhang, M., Huang, G.Q.: IoT and digital twin enabled smart tracking for safety management. Comput. Oper. Res. **128**, 105183 (2021)
67. Liu, Y., Zhang, L., Yang, Y., Zhou, L., Ren, L., Wang, F., Liu, R., Pang, Z., Deen, M.J.: A novel cloud-based framework for the elderly healthcare services using digital twin. IEEE Access **7**, 49088–49101 (2019)
68. Pilati, F., Tronconi, R., Nollo, G., Heragu, S.S., Zerzer, F.: Digital twin of COVID-19 mass vaccination centers. Sustainability **13**(13), 7396 (2021)
69. Barresi, G., Zenzeri, J., Tessadori, J., Laffranchi, M., Semprini, M., Michieli, L.D.: Neurogerontechnologies: applications and opportunities. In: Internet of Things for Human-Centered Design, pp 123–153. Springer (2022)

70. Petrushin, A., Freddolini, M., Barresi, G., Bustreo, M., Laffranchi, M., Bue, A.D., Michieli, L.D.: IoT-Powered monitoring systems for geriatric healthcare: overview. In: Internet of Things for Human-Centered Design, pp. 99–122 (2022)
71. Ackerman, M.J., Filart, R., Burgess, L.P., Lee, I., Poropatich, R.K.: Developing next-generation telehealth tools and technologies: patients, systems, and data perspectives. Telemed. e-Health **16**(1), 93–95 (2010)
72. Tröbinger, M., Costinescu, A., Xing, H., Elsner, J., Hu, T., Naceri, A., Figueredo, L., Jensen, E., Burschka, D., Haddadin, S.: A dual doctor-patient twin paradigm for transparent remote examination, diagnosis, and rehabilitation. In: 2021 IEEE/RSJ International Conference on Intelligent Robots and Systems (IROS). IEEE, pp. 2933–2940 (2021)
73. Benis, A., Tamburis, O., Chronaki, C., Moen, A.: One digital health: a unified framework for future health ecosystems. J. Med. Internet Res. **23**(2), e22189 (2021)
74. Rodríguez-Aguilar, R., Marmolejo-Saucedo, J.-A.: Conceptual framework of digital health public emergency system: digital twins and multiparadigm simulation. EAI Endors. Trans. Pervasive Health Technol. **6**(21), e3–e3 (2020)
75. Laaki, H., Miche, Y., Tammi, K.: Prototyping a digital twin for real time remote control over mobile networks: application of remote surgery. IEEE Access **7**, 20325–20336 (2019)
76. Taylor, L., Dibb, B.: Exploring users and non-users views of the digital twin on a mHealth app: a thematic, qualitative approach. Cogent Psychol. **9**(1), 2079802 (2022)
77. Behm-Morawitz, E.: Mirrored selves: The influence of self-presence in a virtual world on health, appearance, and well-being. Comput. Hum. Behav. **29**(1), 119–128 (2013)
78. Fox, J., Bailenson, J.N., Tricase, L.: The embodiment of sexualized virtual selves: the Proteus effect and experiences of self-objectification via avatars. Comput. Hum. Behav. **29**(3), 930–938 (2013)
79. Wrzesien, M., Rodríguez, A., Rey, B., Alcañiz, M., Baños, R.M., Vara, M.D.: How the physical similarity of avatars can influence the learning of emotion regulation strategies in teenagers. Comput. Hum. Behav. **43**, 101–111 (2015)
80. Horne, M., Hill, A., Murells, T., Ugail, H., Chinnadorai, R., Hardy, M.: Using avatars in weight management settings: a systematic review. Internet Interv. **19**, 100295 (2020)
81. Kim, Y., Sundar, S.S.: Visualizing ideal self vs. actual self through avatars: impact on preventive health outcomes. Comput. Human Behav. **28**(4), 1356–1364 (2012)
82. Matsangidou, M., Otkhmezuri, B., Ang, C.S., Avraamides, M., Riva, G., Gaggioli, A., Iosif, D., Karekla, M.: "Now i can see me" designing a multi-user virtual reality remote psychotherapy for body weight and shape concerns. Human-Comput. Interact. **37**(4), 314–340 (2022)
83. Blut, M., Wang, C., Wünderlich, N.V., Brock, C.: Understanding anthropomorphism in service provision: a meta-analysis of physical robots, chatbots, and other AI. J. Acad. Mark. Sci. **49**(4), 632–658 (2021)
84. Godfrey, S.B., Barresi, G.: Video games for positive aging: playfully engaging older adults. In: Internet of Things for Human-Centered Design, pp. 375–404. Springer (2022)
85. Harichandran, A., Johansen, K.W., Jacobsen, E.L., Teizer, J.: A conceptual framework for construction safety training using dynamic virtual reality games and digital twins. In: ISARC. Proceedings of the International Symposium on Automation and Robotics in Construction. IAARC Publications, pp. 621–628 (2021)
86. El Saddik, A., Badawi, H., Velazquez, R.A.M., Laamarti, F., Diaz, R.G., Bagaria, N., Arteaga-Falconi, J.S.: Dtwins: a digital twins ecosystem for health and well-being. IEEE COMSOC MMTC Commun. Front. **14**, 39–43 (2019)
87. Choukou, M.-A.: Sustainability of mHealth solutions for healthcare system strengthening. In: Digital Health, pp 171–189. Elsevier (2021)
88. Corti, L., Afferni, P., Bertolaso, M.: Healthcare 4.0 and human-centric approach. MEDIC (2020)
89. Afferni, P., Merone, M., Soda, P.: Hospital 4.0 and its innovation in methodologies and technologies. In: 2018 IEEE 31st International Symposium on Computer-Based Medical Systems (CBMS), IEEE, pp 333–338 (2018)

90. Sarangi, S., Choudhury, S.B., Jain, P., Bhatt, P.V., Ramanath, S., Sharma, R., Srinivasu, P.: Development and deployment of a scalable IoT Framework for digital farming applications. In: 2018 IEEE Global Humanitarian Technology Conference (GHTC). IEEE, pp. 1–2 (2018)
91. Gaggioli, A.: Phygital spaces: when atoms meet bits. Cyberpsychol. Behav. Soc. Netw. **20**(12), 774–774 (2017)
92. Soloviov, E., Danilov, A.: The beginning of phygital world. South Asian J. Eng. Technol. **10** (2020)
93. Gregory, D.: Healthcare Goes Digital: Designing for the Convergence of the Digital and Physical Environment—Implications for Design Professionals. SAGE Publications Sage CA, Los Angeles, CA (2022)
94. Yoon, K., Kim, S.-K., Jeong, S.P., Choi, J.-H. Interfacing cyber and physical worlds: introduction to IEEE 2888 standards. In: 2021 IEEE International Conference on Intelligent Reality (ICIR). IEEE, pp 49–50 (2021)
95. Frossard, L., Lloyd, D.: The future of bionic limbs. Res. Features **134**, 74–77 (2021)
96. Chen, D., Ottikkutti, S., Tahmasebi, K.N.: A mechatronics-twin framework based on Stewart platform for effective exploration of operational behaviors of prosthetic sockets with amputees. In: BIODEVICES-16th International Conference on Biomedical Electronics and Devices (2022)
97. Pizzolato, C., Saxby, D.J., Palipana, D., Diamond, L.E., Barrett, R.S., Teng, Y.D., Lloyd, D.G.: Neuromusculoskeletal modeling-based prostheses for recovery after spinal cord injury. Front. Neurorobot. **97** (2019)
98. Wright, J.M., Regele, O.B., Kourtis, L.C., Pszenny, S.M., Sirkar, R., Kovalchick, C., Jones, G.B.: Evolution of the digital biomarker ecosystem. Dig. Med. **3**(4), 154 (2017)
99. Kwok, P.K., Yan, M., Qu, T., Lau, H.Y.: User acceptance of virtual reality technology for practicing digital twin-based crisis management. Int. J. Comput. Integr. Manuf. **34**(7–8), 874–887 (2021)
100. Leo, C.G., Tumolo, M.R., Sabina, S., Colella, R., Recchia, V., Ponzini, G., Fotiadis, D.I., Bodini, A., Mincarone, P.: Health technology assessment for in silico medicine: social, ethical and legal aspects. Int. J. Environ. Res. Public Health **19**(3), 1510 (2022)
101. Huang, P.-H., Kim, K.-H., Schermer, M.: Ethical issues of digital twins for personalized health care service: preliminary mapping study. J. Med. Internet Res. **24**(1), e33081 (2022)
102. Nyholm, S.: Should a medical digital twin be viewed as an extension of the patient's body? J. Med. Ethics **47**(6), 401–402 (2021)
103. Bruynseels, K., Santoni de Sio, F., Van den Hoven, J.: Digital twins in health care: ethical implications of an emerging engineering paradigm. Front. Genet. **31** (2018)
104. Braun, M.: Represent me: please! towards an ethics of digital twins in medicine. J. Med. Ethics **47**(6), 394–400 (2021)
105. Nurgalieva, L., O'Callaghan, D., Doherty, G.: Security and privacy of mHealth applications: a scoping review. IEEE Access **8**, 104247–104268 (2020)
106. Perno, M., Hvam, L., Haug, A.: Enablers and barriers to the implementation of digital twins in the process industry: a systematic literature review. In: 2020 IEEE International Conference on Industrial Engineering and Engineering Management (IEEM). IEEE, pp 959–964 (2020)
107. Yi, C., Park, S., Yang, C., Jiang, F., Ding, Z., Zhu, J., Liu, J.: Muscular human cybertwin for internet of everything: a pilot study. IEEE Trans. Ind. Inf. (2022)

# mHealth for Well-Being: Case Studies in Physiological, Cognitive, and Affective Sensing

**Sachin Patel, Mayuri Duggirala, Avik Ghose, and Aniruddha Sinha**

## 1 Introduction

Mobile health (mHealth) is defined by the World Health Organization's (WHO) Global Observatory for eHealth (GOe) as "*medical and public health practice supported by mobile devices, such as mobile phones, patient monitoring devices, personal digital assistants (PDAs), and other wireless devices*" [1]. A primary motive for the creation of mHealth solutions has been its ability to substitute or complement medical advice when it is not available. mHealth solutions can leverage the device computing power to provide features based on Artificial Intelligence, mobile sensors, and immersive experiences. Needless to mention the benefits of so-called "digital" technologies, such as scalability, accessibility, connectivity, and availability. The WHO GOe has surveyed categories of mHealth services and 14 categories have been identified, namely, health call centers, emergency toll-free telephone services, managing emergencies and disasters, mobile telemedicine, appointment reminders, community mobilization and health promotion, treatment compliance, mobile patient records, information access, patient monitoring, health surveys and data collection, surveillance, health awareness raising, and decision support systems [1].

S. Patel (✉) · M. Duggirala
TCS Research, Tata Consultancy Services Ltd., Pune, India
e-mail: sachin.patel@tcs.com

M. Duggirala
e-mail: mayuri.duggirala@tcs.com

A. Ghose · A. Sinha
TCS Research, Tata Consultancy Services Ltd., Kolkata, India
e-mail: avik.ghose@tcs.com

A. Sinha
e-mail: aniruddha.s@tcs.com

 
S. Scataglini et al. (eds.), *mHealth and Human-Centered Design Towards Enhanced Health, Care, and Well-Being*, Studies in Big Data 120,
https://doi.org/10.1007/978-981-99-3989-3_5

In this chapter, we present two mHealth case studies, first one being a mobile stress management solution and the second one being a mobile and wearable-based cognitive analysis solution. We begin the chapter with a summary of key concerns in building mHealth solutions for well-being/mental health. These concerns/challenges are distilled from our experience working on the two case studies and are meant to serve as a guide for those building such solutions.

Mental illness impacts a large portion of the population, and the problem is growing. In any given year, 1 in 5 adults has a mental illness—impacting not only those 52.9 million (2020 statistic) people but also their family, friends, colleagues, and communities. [2] The overall growth is largely driven by higher rates of mental illness in 18 to 25-year-olds [2]. Mental illness and chronic illness often co-occur, complicating the treatment for both. People with both chronic illness and behavioral health conditions have costs higher than those with only chronic illness. Another pressing issue is that of access to treatment. According to WHO Mental Health Atlas 2014, more than 45% of the world population lives in a country where there is less than 1 psychiatrist for every 100,000 people [3]. Relying solely on specialists to provide services for people affected by mental health problems would prevent millions of people from accessing the services they need. Addressing treatment gaps will be key as the disparity in demand and supply widens. Today, treatment gaps persist due to stigma and difficulty accessing treatment. Closing treatment gaps will require solutions to address workforce shortages. As per projections for 2030, demand will exceed supply and result in excessive shortage of mental health professionals [4]. Mobile Health solutions can scale (addresses workforce shortage), are accessible (eliminates location constraints), and can provide treatment in a privacy-protected manner (addresses the stigma issue). mHealth, thus, offers a compelling value proposition with respect to addressing many of the constraints in mental health treatment.

## 2 Challenges in Mobile Mental Health

In this section, we present the key concerns in the making of a mobile mental health solution. Following this section, we shall present a case study of the making of a mobile stress management solution and our experience with addressing some of these concerns.

### *2.1 Sensing and Assessment*

Mental health misdiagnosis is an alarmingly prevalent phenomenon that keeps you from being able to achieve psychological wellness. A 2009 meta-analysis of 50,000 patients published in the Lancet found that general practitioners only correctly identified depression in patients in 47.3% of cases [5]. This keeps people from receiving the right treatment, resulting in further distress, and could threaten emotional and behavioral function of the individual. The advances in speech, vision, and language AI as well as sensing technology have opened up an opportunity for addressing some of the concerns in mental health assessment. The ubiquity of smartphones and wearables makes it possible to measure and analyze a wide range of behaviors, some examples being affective states, physical activity, social connectedness, contextual factors, social media behaviors, physiological markers and sleep behaviors. A constant challenge in many of the mental health assessment questionnaires is the bias. There have been evidences of racial biases affecting assessment. The study proposed in [6] presents evidence on bias found in assessing people of different colors. The recency bias, which means that while the patient might have good memory of the last few days, it is hard for the patient to recollect experiences/behaviors exhibited over last few months (most patients do not meet the practitioners more frequently than that). To address this concern, the behavior monitoring technology can be leveraged to augment the counselor's assessment process with reliable and longitudinal behavioral data.

## 2.2 Design and Engagement

mHealth solutions provide an accessible and scalable route for delivering evidence-based psychotherapy protocols to those in need. However, most apps suffer from low user retention rates when released in the wild. Across a sample of 93 mental health apps (with median total installs of 100,000), median Day-N retention rates at 15-day and 30-day stages were only 3.9% (IQR 10.3%) and 3.3% (IQR 6.2%), respectively [7]. People with mental health issues such as depression are characterized by persistently sad moods, lack of interest, low motivation, and unlikely to stay engaged. Most therapies are long term and effective treatment would require patients to complete the recommended duration of therapy. More so, in order to leverage the newer advances in AI/sensing, it is necessary for users to use the apps for longer periods of time to help the AI learn better and make more accurate predictions.

## 2.3 Interventions—Identification, Contextualization, and Digitization

According to WHO Mental Health Atlas 2014, more than 45% of the world population lives in a country where there is less than 1 psychiatrist for every 100,000 people [3]. Relying solely on specialists to provide services for people affected by mental health problems would prevent millions of people from accessing the services they need. A meta-analysis showed that up to 38% of Major Depressive Episodes (MDE) could be prevented with currently available interventions [8]. This indicates that there is immense value to be unlocked from the existing evidence on intervention efficacy. The mHealth community has an opportunity to operationalize such interventions that have strong/high-quality evidence and make them accessible to the population.

## 2.4 Data Privacy and the Security versus Usability Trade-Off

The negative attitude towards mental health and the associated stigma are significant hurdles in the willingness of people to seek treatment [9]. It is hence critical to assure users of the confidentiality and privacy of their data. Any kind of disclosure of mental health status is likely to affect the user in multiple ways such as—avoidance of care, denial of certain services, and discrimination by their employers/colleagues. mHealth solutions need to be cognizant of the fact that while utmost regard is given to these aspects, there may be conditions, e.g., suicidal tendencies, where the caregiver or the counselor must be notified of patient status. The trade-off between security and usability has been widely discussed in the literature. This becomes a crucial issue, given that mobile mental health apps have already been suffering from low user retention rates. The privacy and security strategies must be designed appropriately with respect to the condition being treated and the sensitivity of the data being collected.

## 2.5 Digital Platform for Data Management

A data management platform helps collect and analyze large amount of data. Health data are characterized by high sensitivity and special regulatory requirements. Healthcare industry regulations such as Health Insurance Portability and Accountability Act (HIPAA) [10] require that data be protected with audit trail, data encryption, SSL for data transfer, and role-based access. Similarly, there is a need to adhere to data protection regulations such as the General Data Protection Regulation (GDPR) [11]. Such regulations would require aspects such as consent, transparency in data processing, user's rights w.r.t. control over own data, data privacy strategies to be in place. Many regulations are geography-specific, and the data management platform must support all such requirements. Data Analysis in such a platform would have multiple aims, such as to discover population level patterns to assist stakeholder with decision-making, to identify individual level anomalies (without identifying the individual), and enhance the AI systems for making better predictions.

## 2.6 Ethics and Safety

Amongst ethical considerations, a critical concern is that of corporates misusing sensitive data for surveillance and discrimination. Mental health data are particularly prone to such misuse. The data protection and health data regulations do help address this issue to a certain extent. However, these regulations may not be able to stop app makers from developing features like targeted advertising, which is based on individual's personal data and may create an environment of distrust. While an app may take all necessary permissions to collect certain data, there usually is no way for the user to know what data are necessary for the features she needs to use. Furthermore, the user is the one who has a pressing need to receive the treatment, hence the user has no choice but to agree to whatever permissions the app is seeking. The onus, thus, is on app makers to follow ethical design principles in such matters. Safety and accountability are other crucial aspects given the possibility of self-harm by vulnerable users and resulting litigation against the app maker. Many apps found on app stores are not necessarily built on strong evidence and are likely to cause adverse effects. People in difficult circumstances are attracted by such inexpensive solutions and may end up worsening their own condition. The need for the FDA or other centralized body to coordinate the systematic gathering of data on possible adverse effects of digital mental health tools has been emphasized in the literature [12].

## 2.7 Validation/Trials and Long Cycle Time to Market

The validation process for mHealth solutions is a long one comprising of iterative testing of design prototypes, independent validation of interventions, sensors and AI models, functional and non-functional (performance and usability) testing, clinical trials, and pilot testing in the wild. Each step is likely to result in further iterations in the cycle. Furthermore, the solution is likely to show unexpected results once deployed in the wild and could result in a lot of reworks. Depending on the claims made by the solution provider, the enforcement authorities would require that sufficient good quality evidence is produced. Often, multiple trials are required before the claim can be substantiated. Identifying the right partner for the clinical trials and later stages is critical. Mental health treatment service providers, medical colleges, and hospitals could all be potential partners.

## 2.8 Adoption by Practitioner Community

The field of healthcare is naturally resistant to change due to the risk involved. In the area of mental health, this is further pronounced because its users are vulnerable and unpredictable, due to which practitioners find comfort in tried and tested methods and are likely to hesitate in trying something new. While most practitioners are trained on the evidence-based practices in their field, their training usually does not include the new evidence being generated in the digital sphere. This limits their awareness, which is also a significant hurdle in mHealth adoption. There is also a fear within the practitioners that such mHealth solutions are being made to automate or take away their jobs. This further adds to the resistance. At time, the technologies themselves may not be up to the mark. Past experiences with mHealth solutions, wearables, sensors etc. have shown that while they demonstrate excellent results in the studies, clinical trials (controlled environments), they do not necessarily perform as well in the wild. Such a gap creates distrust in the evidence and mHealth solutions in general [13].

## 3 Case Study I—A Mobile Stress Management Solution

In this section, we present our experience with developing and deploying a mobile-based stress management solution to be used by associates in an IT services organization. The app aims at periodically assessing factors such as emotions, stress, productivity and provides interventions for instant stress relief as well as building stress immunity over a period.

### *3.1 Sensing Stress and Emotions*

A multi-pronged strategy for sensing emotions and stress has been employed in the app. This comprises daily probes (single question scales), validated assessment scales, AI-based methods such as emotion recognition from voice, stress detection from mobile sensors, and stress and sentiment recognition from textual journal entries.

#### 3.1.1 Emotion Recognition from Voice

Emotions play a significant role in human life experience and decision-making and are known to influence a variety of workplace factors such as engagement, productivity, and overall well-being. Thus, measuring emotions is an essential feature of this solution. We express emotions through speech and hence audio signals are an excellent data source to analyze emotions. This option is attractive also because of its non-obtrusive nature and ubiquity of microphones in smartphones. A machine learning model based on para-linguistic features of audio streams was developed. This model classifies emotions into three affect classes of positive, neutral, and negative. Unlike most publicly available emotion datasets which have acted data, speech in the workplace is more subtle in nature, hence the public datasets were not suitable for the training task. To address this issue, an emotion induction procedure was designed and executed to generate a dataset of non-acted speech data. Following this, an exploratory analysis of various speech feature sets and machine learning techniques helped us to arrive at the best model fit. The models demonstrated an emotion classification accuracy of 73%, which exceeds the accuracies reported in literature for non-acted speech for a speaker-dependent test set. The performance of the same model was tested on the public dataset Emo-DB, and we found the speaker-dependent recognition accuracy to be around 95% [14, 15].

#### 3.1.2 Mobile Sensor-Based Stress Predictor

With a goal of generating a mobile-sensor dataset, we developed an Android mobile app that logs sensor data while also periodically asking the user to report her stress levels, using a single question probe. Primarily sensors related to mobile usage, ambient light, accelerometer, power on/off times, etc. were logged. 30 subjects in an educational institute were asked to use the app over a period of 15 days. The sensor dataset, thus, generated along with ground truth (self-reported stress levels) was used to train an AI model that could predict stress levels. Both traditional machine learning techniques (support vector machines, k-nearest neighbor, decision trees) and deep learning techniques (deep neural networks) were explored. The KNN model showed the best accuracy of 76% in classifying stress vs no stress classes. The model is now integrated into the stress management mobile app and we hope that accuracies will improve over time as we obtain more data.

#### 3.1.3 Sentiment and Stress Recognition from Textual Journal Entries

The practice of writing daily journals is a widely acknowledged well-being intervention, as it promotes self-awareness and helps cope with emotional disturbances. An analysis of such journal entries could lead to deeper insights into well-being of individuals by way of extracting insights such as mentions of stress, sentiments, and sources of the sentiment. We employed Natural Language Processing and deep learning techniques (ensemble models using Bi-LSTM and RNN) to detect, extract, and classify author's activity phrases and sentiments from the journal texts. The automatic extraction of self-reported activities could be done with a precision of 92.84% and recall of 71.8% and classification of the extracted activities with an overall 70.16% precision and 76.6% recall. Sentiment classification in three classes of positive, negative, and neutral gave an accuracy of 79.56%. These models were trained on elaborate datasets sourced from a variety of datasets like Twitter, airline reviews, HappyDB, Twitter new year resolutions and our own data collection for journal entries [16]. A model to recognize if stress has been expressed was also built with the Twitter data. The data were classified into four classes of critical stress, stress, no stress, and eustress. Post the labeling process, we did not find a good balance within various classes, hence we reduced the annotations to two classes of "stress" and "no stress". A deep learning architecture comprising of LSTM + RNN model with softmax layer was employed to create the classifier. We got 81% of validation accuracy and on our journal dataset, and we got around 78% test accuracy on predicting stress/no stress. All these models, namely, sentiment, stress, activity extraction, activity classification have been integrated into the journaling feature of the app and visualizations based on the insights are presented to users in a timeline view.

**Probes and Assessment Scales**

Probes are single question instruments that help understand specific aspects of user's states with minimal investment of time. The app has many such probes embedded within the overall experience. For example, at the start of the day, a question "*A new day is about to begin. Would you like to reflect on how you are feeling right now?*" is asked, whereas towards the end of the day a question "*As you are about to end your work day, would you like to take a minute and tell us how you are feeling right now?*" is asked. Some probes also aim at understanding the effectiveness of certain interventions. For example, one of the questions that pops up after playing a stressbuster game is "*I was able to restart my work with better focus after I played with the stressbuster*". We have relied on such probes throughout the app primarily because the longer multi-question instruments take more time and users are likely to skip them or just click any option because they are bored of doing it. The cognitive effort involved in responding to these single question probes is much lesser and we can hope to get good quality data. Having said that the importance of using the gold standard instruments cannot be undermined. We also have an assessment module with the app where such scales have been made available and users are nudged to periodically assess themselves on these. For example, the Perceived Stress Scale is a validated and popular scale that is part of the assessment module [17].

## *3.2 Interventions for Stress Management*

The team of psychologists inspects the behavioral sciences literature to identify the interventions that hold strong evidence and are also amenable to digitization and self-administration through a digital app. The focus is on identifying behavioral interventions that do not need clinical/professional guidance for administration. Some examples of interventions that have been designed and implemented so far include:

- Guided deep breathing sessions.
- Mindfulness activities such as mindful walking and eating.
- Sleep regulation—guides the user into a better sleep routine.
- Cognitive restructuring—help the user identify and classify distorted thoughts and help in a changed/improved outlook.
- Journaling—Describing daily experience and help users self-reflect. Also assisted by an AI-based analysis of the textual diary entries.

- Games to deliver laughter therapy, color therapy, and music therapy.
- Stress relief interventions such as plan the day, jot down positive thoughts, express gratitude, get better hydration, etc.

The process of intervention identification may involve meta-analysis of existing evidence to choose the ones with the strongest effect size. Many interventions are designed and validated in different cultures and may need some degree of contextualization while being operationalized. Where necessary the intervention may need independent studies to validate their effects after digitization. The overall organization and delivery of interventions is guided by our ABC Intervention Framework. This framework ensures that each wellness package has an activity to address the three aspects of Affect, Behavior, and Cognition, thus ensuring completeness of the intervention approach.

### *3.3 Design Strategies*

The app is designed for the working age population and its features are designed with the specific cohort in mind. This includes strategies such as:

- **Companion App with Digital Pet**: The user interacts with a pet character (dog) throughout the app experience. The visuals of the pet create a feeling of trustworthiness and warmth, which are characteristics of a dog. The app also attempts to build trust, by reminding the user of how its recommendations are based on strong evidence from the literature.
- **Serious games**: These are games with a purpose in addition to entertainment. Examples of designs we have employed include stress buster games such as ColorMe that engages users in a game where throwing colored balloons on a blank painting imparts colors to different parts of the painting [18]. An example of a digitized mental health intervention is a whale swimming in the sea and the user is expected to match his breathing pattern with the movement of the whale. While providing a game like experience, this also serves as a stress relief intervention.
- **Sensor-based games/interactions**: We have designed novel interactions that leverage the sensing capability available in mobile devices. This is done by leveraging specific mobile sensing capability to control games. For example, in a laughter-based game, the user is shown a wilted flower on the screen and the goal of the game is to laugh out loud. As the user laughs the flower begins to bloom, the end goal of the game being a fully bloomed flower. The game not only provides stress relief through laughter therapy but also makes for a highly interactive user experience [19]. Another example is a blow-based game where the user is required to blow away clouds on the screen by blowing into the microphone. This provides a deep breathing intervention, while playing the game [20].
- **Playful interactions**: A typical transactional task on user interfaces can get boring if performed repeatedly. With a goal of sustaining the user's curiosity, mini games

have been designed, which are not necessarily features visible to the user but surprise the user once in a while. For example, a cluttered screen with garbage spread on the screen pops-up and user is challenged to drag all pieces into a trash can. Another example is of a mood tracking feature where users could get bored reporting on a Likert scale all too often. This interface is replaced with a slider which can be dragged to modify a scenery on the screen. The two ends of the scale are contrasted as greenery on one end and a desert on the other. As the users moves the slider to indicate his mood, the scenery changes from greenery to desert and vice versa. This makes the boring task of reporting moods, engaging, and playful.

## 3.4 Privacy and Security Strategies

We have followed a privacy by design approach while designing the app, with basic principles of the GDPR being the guiding principles [11]. The app does not collect any personally identifiable data. Even for the user id, we prompt the users to choose a pseudonym instead of using their real name. This is done so that the app gains trust of the user and the user does not hesitate to share any kind of data with the system. Data such as entries in the daily journal, where free flowing text entry is possible, are encrypted in the system to prohibit any kind of data exposure. The app gives the users full control over their data by enabling them to download a digital copy of the data, withdraw from the data collection at any point as well as completely purge all data in the system. For security, we use a token-based authentication system where the token would expire periodically, after which the user would be prompted to login again using the user id and password. The Forget password feature is based on five security questions. We have avoided collecting email addresses or mobile numbers at all places so as to assure users that it is impossible for the system to know their identity.

## 3.5 Data Management Platform

The Data Management Platform (DMP) is based on a microservice architecture with most of its services exposed as REST APIs. This enables easy integration with the front-end apps or any other solution that could benefit from the features of the DMP.

The key components of the DMP are shown in Fig. 1. The functions of these components are as follows:

- **Engage**—Users of the platform interact with the system through the Engage layer. This comprises of the mobile app and a web portal. The web portal enables users to view their personal dashboards based on data collected by the app. If more such apps are integrated with the system (say for example a physical fitness app)

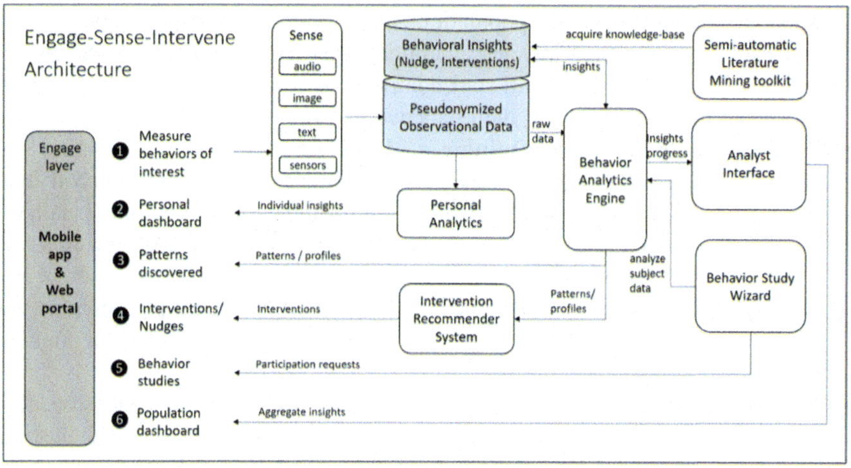


**Fig. 1** Data management platform

both the data sources (stress management and physical fitness) could be used to present a unified view on the portal.

- **Sense**—The various sensing AI models are bundled in this component. Each model is exposed as a REST API that can be invoked from the mobile app.
- **Pseudonymized data store**—Users of the app login with pseudonyms and the app does not collect any personally identifiable data. These data comprise of various sensed states as well as a log of activities performed by the user.
- **Personal Analytics**—The user gets to see visualizations of his personal data with insights generated by this component.
- **Analyst Interface**—The portal also has a provision for other user types such as Human Resources and Behavioral scientists. These users get to see aggregate dashboards of the population data. The data being generated by various behavior studies rolled out on the platform are made accessible over the analyst interface. The mode of operation here is that analysts do not get to download any of the data but are only able to upload their data processing algorithms to the system and view the insights being generated.
- **Behavior Analytics Engine**—This component analyzes the observational data to discover patterns of interest. This feature works in conjunction with the Intervention recommender module where healthy and unhealthy patterns in emotion data are discovered and sent to the Recommender for identification of an appropriate intervention.
- **Behavior Study Wizard**—The behavior study wizard contains a workflow to design and publish studies. Most features of this module are accessible to the Behavioral Scientist role. The Scientist would first design a study as a part of which she would need to also specify all the variables to be measured in the study. Each variable would be associated with a corresponding measurement tool and the app from which the data are to be collected. Once the study is designed, the

scientist will publish it to the population. At this point, all users of the apps will get a notification about the study and an option to participate. The users who choose to participate in the study will start contributing their data to the study and the Scientists will start receiving their data over the Analysts Interface.

- **Semi-automatic literature mining toolkit**—The behavior science literature holds a wealth of knowledge, especially the empirical research, which if digitized can be leveraged in multiple ways. For example, digitizing and visualizing relationships between different variables at play in a certain phenomenon will help behavior scientists get an overall view of the current research and derive new hypothesis for studies. We have developed a set of NLP and AI programs that semi-automatically mine the literature to discover empirical results and populate the behavioral insights data store.
- **Behavioral Insights data store**—This is a behavioral knowledge data store. The knowledge is stored in the form of relations between variables along with the relation type (correlation, causation) and other relation parameters such as strength. Other kind of data in this store is that of Interventions. A structure has been designed to hold complete data about an Intervention and is entered manually by the behavioral scientist. In case the data are obtained semi-automatically from the literature mining toolkit, the knowledge management interface is used to curate the data and ensure that only valid entries go into the system.
- **Intervention Recommender**—The intervention recommender works based on the curated intervention repository, which is part of the behavioral insights data store. Through this module, Behavior Scientists maintain a mapping between patterns and interventions. When the Behavior Analytics engine discovers a pattern in the observational data, the corresponding intervention is picked from the repository and pushed to the delivery channel chosen for the intervention. A delivery channel could be an app activity and notification message.

### *3.6 Validation and Pilot Studies*

A multi-pronged validation strategy was adopted to validate the app and its capabilities. These included expert reviews, community forums, design observational studies, focus groups as well as large-scale rollouts.

- **Expert reviews and community forums**—The overall approach and feature set was presented to team of experts in mental health ranging from psychiatrists and psychotherapists with several decades of clinical experience, as well as with end users from various contexts such as organizations, healthcare, and academia. Early versions of the work were also presented at specialized conferences with a focus on mental health, psychiatry, and psychological counseling and therapy.
- **Design feedback and observational studies**—Design feedback by users from our focus groups and beta users was taken periodically. In one such exercise, we gave the app to a batch of associates newly joining the organization and

asked them to use the app for a week. Following this, an open house people was organized, where we asked to share features, they liked or disliked. With another smaller group of users (seven members), we conducted an observational study in which users were asked to use the app in a closed room with a designer making observations about where users get stuck or take time to understand a feature. For design aspects too we got expert feedback from accomplished designers, which helped refine the designs.

- **Validation of the Artificial Intelligence features**—The AI features have a validation and test cycle of their own. We ensured that we train our models on data that is very similar to the target data on which the prediction is to be made. For this, an emotion induction data collection study (33 subjects) and a daily journal study were conducted with the organization (250 subjects). These datasets were used to train the voice emotion and journal sentiment models, respectively. The real test of the models, however, will be in the wild where data are likely to be sparse and more varied. In our pilot rollouts, we did not see much usage of these features, hence we await larger scale rollouts to validate the models.
- **Efficacy of the app**—We carried out three studies for 632 users in a large global IT services organization who used the app between January and August 2020, using a mixed methods approach surveys, interviews, and focus groups. While a lot of design and app-related feedback was obtained, the primary motive was to substantiate our claim that "*the app reduces stress*". While a few users did use the app for the full duration and reducing trends in their stress levels were noticed, we were unable to get statistically significant results due to sparse usage data. These studies were followed by a large-scale rollout of the app across the India division of the organization. Over 900 + users downloaded the app. Since it was a partial functionality app, the users did not have much motive to use the app beyond the first week, hence we were not able to compare the drop-out rates with the benchmarks and the usage duration was too small to draw conclusions on stress reduction. Next, we plan to conduct randomized controlled trials and large-scale rollouts with a full-featured version of the app.

## 4 Case Study II—A Cognitive Analysis Application

In this section, we present the effect of cognition on mental health, especially for the anxiety, boredom, and the stress levels during performance of a task. Some of the essential cognitive factors are briefly described followed by few standard methods for measuring the same. The changes in cognitive load during a task gets reflected in physiology and the same can be measured using wearable sensors. We present few studies on measuring such physiological changes and their relationship with the stress and anxiety, which are the key factors in determining the condition of the mental health.

## 4.1 Importance of Cognitive Analysis in Mental Health

Cognitive load is quantified as the volume of mental resources required for processing any information or to perform any task. John Sweller first introduced the concept of cognitive load theory [21] in late 1980s. This theory was built based on Atkinson's model of human information processing [22]. According to this model, there are primarily three types of memory, namely, sensory, short-term, and long-term memory. The information received from sensory memory are passed to short- and long-term memory for processing. Baddeley [23] proposed the model of working memory, which describes the principle of the short-term memory. The amount of working memory [21] used during processing of a task in the brain provides a measure of the cognitive load for that task. Working memory is believed to have limited capacity and hence is vulnerable to overload. Hence, the effectiveness of a task depends on the amount of cognitive load experienced by a subject.

The performance of an individual for a given task depends on the individual cognitive skill and the challenge associated with the task. If the skill level is quite low compared to the given challenge, then one experiences anxiety. On the contrary, if the challenge is low compared to the skill, then one tends to get bored. While performing a task, whenever there is a balance between the challenge and the individual's ability/skill, then the experience is described as the Flow state [24]. In this state, an individual is fully involved in the task without any distractions [25]. High cognitive load, in a task, affects the performance. Hence, in general, it is vital to analyze and quantify the cognitive load that would be experienced for a given task.

The mental state of an individual depends on how comfortable is an individual while performing various tasks in the daily living scenario. The change in mental state could happen due to the amount of imparted cognitive load, anxiety, boredom, etc. If the cognitive load experience by an individual goes beyond a critical point [22], then the performance of the subject may deteriorate drastically. Thus, it is always required to maintain an optimal level of cognitive load to increase the efficiency, which would also enable for a good mental health.

## 4.2 Cognitive Factors

According to Sweller [21], there are three types of cognitive load [26], namely, Intrinsic, Extraneous, and Germane. Each of these types affects the performance of an individual during a learning and decision-making process. They are briefly described below:

- **Intrinsic load**—This is the inherent difficulty level associated with a particular task or some learning topic. It refers to the complexity of the task.
- **Extraneous load**—This load reflects the difficulty level in understanding an information due to the way it is represented to the learner.

- **Germane load**—This is generated due to processing and construction of schema. It helps in learning a new technology.

Intrinsic load is believed to be unchangeable, but extraneous and germane load can be manipulated by instructors in order to achieve a better and fruitful learning experience. It is always desirable to reduce the Extraneous load while promoting the Germane load [27]. In the present research work, we focus on the evaluation of the Intrinsic load for a textual content. In general, the cognitive load is affected by multiple neuropsychological factors, namely, memory, anxiety, boredom, cognitive flow, attention, engagement, perceptual span, etc. Some of these are briefly described below.

- ***Memory***: As mentioned earlier, during performing a task, working memory or short-term memory plays an important role in the experience of cognitive load [21]. The effect of declarative and non-declarative memories, on the performance of real-life tasks, plays a very critical role [28]. These include episodic memory (dealing with various activities of an individual in the past), semantic memory (dealing with acquisition and remembering about rules, facts, associations, knowledge, which are generic and not related to any specific task), implicit memory (where the actual learning episode is unaware of), procedural memory (related to skills and habits), and verbal memory (related to words and abstractions from language). Additionally, there are memories associated with various sensory inputs, namely, auditory, visual, proprioceptive, tactile, and olfactory [29]. Each of these types of memories affects the cognition in a diverse manner, hence the analysis of the same is quite complex. In the present research work, the effect of semantic and verbal memory related to language processing is expected to be reflected in the electrophysiology-based cognitive analysis.
- ***Cognitive Flow***: Cognitive and emotional states are the outcome of individual skill and challenge level of the task. Low (high) skill and high (low) challenge result into a state of anxiety (boredom) [30]. When skill and challenge match, a state of focused concentration and enjoyment is attained. This is termed as Flow state or Cognitive Flow [24]. Such state is desired for proper learning [31].
- ***Attention***: While performing a task, the level of attention determines the performance of an individual. Experiments on eye gaze movement are done to model the attention during a reading process [32]. During this process, many times, the eye gaze remains fairly static for approximately 250 ms, which is termed as fixation [33]. Shift in the eye gaze for successive fixations is found to be related to the speed of lexical processing. Attention to a particular word and then subsequent shift to a later word reflects the amount of semantic processing done during the reading [34]. In addition to the eye gaze analysis, the attention affects the engagement of an individual in a task. This gets reflected in the brain signals [35]. Various sensory modes of attention exist, namely, visual, auditory, and spatial [36]. Following the Posner cueing paradigm, the effect of inter-modal cues is found to be linked to the attention, in the detection, localization, and discrimination tasks [37, 38].
- ***Perceptual span***: The amount of spatial information, that is captured during an eye gaze fixation, is termed as the visual field [39]. During a reading task, the

amount of texts read within a visual field, towards the left and right of a fixation is called the perceptual span [40]. This perceptual span gets affected due to change in attention. Hence, analyzing the change in perceptual span provides information on the variation in the attention during a task. It also provides information about the cognitive flow.

## 4.3 Reflection in Physiology

Mental state and mental load have strong correlation in physiological bio-signals. Jaiswal et al. [41] show how mental state can affect heart rate and breathing rate. Rakshit et al. [42] show how heart-rate variability (HRV) correlates with emotional state. Hence, physiological proxies can be used for mental state assessment. This serves as an enabler for using mHealth technologies in the domain of mental well-being monitoring be in stress or mental workload [43].

## 4.4 Standard Measurement/Assessment Methods

There are primarily two standard approaches, for measuring the cognitive load as given below:

- The mental workload can be qualitatively measured using self-reports [30] through semi-structured interviews and questionnaires. Flow state scale is designed by Jackson and Marsh [44] to evaluate flow using feedback questionnaire-based method. User experience is described using flow state questionnaires/scales, which are used to measure both the stress level and performance. In the daily living scenario, the flow and other states of consciousness are measured using experience sampling method, which attempts to capture the key events associated to such mental states. Due to the inherent bias, these feedback and questionnaire-based approaches are not reliable though they seem to be feasible and less complex in nature.
- Objective or causal methods are based on the measurement of physiological changes or behavioral changes. This includes directly measuring the brain activities using functional magnetic resonance imaging (fMRI) [45], functional near infra-red imaging (fNIR) [46], and Electroencephalogram (EEG) [47]. Pupillary response is another means of directly measuring the effect due to brain functions, as the eye gaze and pupil dilation are controlled by cranial nerves [48]. Attempts have been carried out for measuring the cognitive load, using other physiological changes due to sympathetic and para-sympathetic nervous system, like cardiovascular changes [49], galvanic skin resistance [50], photoplethysmogram (PPG) [31].

## 4.5 Wearable-Based Methods

Wearable devices provide a wealth of information about the general health and activity of a user [51]. They provide information like heart rate and breathing rate even in ambulatory conditions [52]. While these have been used primarily for understanding physical health conditions like cardiac disorders [53] or neuro-motor condition [54]. However, HRV, HR, and breathing rate computed from these devices can be utilized for mental wellness [41–43, 51, 52].

One of the case studies in [50], which involves using a wearable device for remote monitoring of mental effort, for example, allows a remote user to monitor the mental effort of a person undertaking a task, using a mobile application (app). This can be used for three purposes:

1. To understand the complexity of a task, given a number of users undertaking the same task and also complex sub-tasks of a given larger tasks.
2. To understand the relative performance of similar users across a task to understand relative strengths and weaknesses of participants.
3. Longitudinal analysis of an individual across tasks and over time to record progress on a particular domain.

Such apps can be used in the domain of education for content analysis and also student stratification. Furthermore, it can be used in workplace for role fitment purposes to avoid burnout and boredom. Such an app clearly illustrates the power of mHealth technologies in the sphere of mental well-being and wellness.

Similarly, [51] provides a method to monitor activity levels using a wearable and connects to a mobile device. Activity levels can also provide useful insights into the physical and mental well-being of the subjects and in case the user is not performing the recommended/expected amount of activity, appropriate nudges to influence the user behavior.

Other technologies like mobile camera-based pupil monitoring [55] may be able to provide cognitive load accurately, however, they are not suited for continuous measurement and estimation. Pramanik et al. [56] provide an extensive review of mobile and wearable technologies in use for physical and mental health monitoring and assessment. The work also indicates that future of wearable sensing is nano-sensors capable of sensing biomarkers from human body. Krishnan et al. [57] illustrate how wellness is multi-dimensional and holistic wellness comes through taking care of both physical and mental well-being in a single model. This kind of multi-modal continuous data can be only obtained via the use of wearable sensors. Mobile applications built using such data are not only used to understand the mental condition but also used to provide real-time feedback/interventions to individuals, as a virtual companion, in order to improve mental health. A typical wearable-based setup for mHealth is shown in Fig. 2.

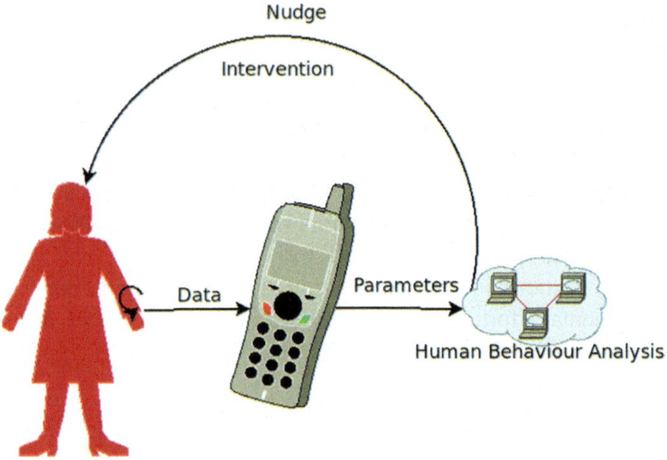


**Fig. 2** Wearable deployment scenario

## 5 Conclusions

We presented a summary of key concerns in building mHealth apps, based on the experience of developing two mHealth solutions, first one being a mobile-based stress management solution and the second one being a wearable-based cognitive analysis solution. The key concerns/challenges presented are specifically in the context of creating mHealth solutions for mental health and well-being. These are sensing and assessment, design and engagement, intervention discovery and operationalization, data privacy and security, ethics and safety, data management platforms, validation and trials, and the resulting long cycle time and adoption by the practitioner community.

The mobile-based stress management solution comprises of a multimodal approach to behavioral assessment and sensing that addresses the limitations of standardized behavioral assessment as well as sensing. In doing so, the proposed solution can leverage the capabilities of sensing technologies from mobiles, while providing contextually rich and realistic data. In creating a privacy preserving solution, we showcase how the proposed solution adheres to industry best practices in recommendations for privacy management for users and is thus ready to meet the needs of privacy sensitive users aiming to interact with the stress management app. Integrating insights from behavioral sciences assessment and interventions, multimodal sensing and serious games, we present a solution that is evidence-based, capable of analyzing behavior in context and provide a playful and engaging yet theoretically grounded solution that can address the needs of users aiming to manage their mental health, their caregivers, and the larger provider ecosystem.

The wearable-based solution presents novel ways to measure well-being factors including cognitive and physiological phenomena such as attention, heart rate, heart rate variability, breathing rate, physical activity to name a few. In the traditional approaches, the cognitive factors are measured using questionnaire-based scoring methods, which provides an indication of the mental health of an individual. The recent advancement of sensing technologies in mobile devices and wearables, it has been possible to understand daily living activities, behavior, measures some of the physiological responses in affordable and unobtrusive manner. Wearables, in conjunction with smartphone-based apps and traditional validated behavioral assessment instruments together, can provide rich insights into well-being and help deliver personalized interventions to the users.

While the technologies continue to mature, these case studies show that an ideal solution would need a truly multi-disciplinary effort. There is a need for designers, policymakers, regulatory entities, technology providers, health practitioners to make concerted efforts to address the various challenges discussed in this chapter.

## References

1. mHealth—New horizons for health through mobile technologies, In: Global Observatory for eHealth Series – Vol. 3. WHO Library. ISBN 978 92 4 156425 0
2. National Institute of Mental Health. https://www.nimh.nih.gov/health/statistics/mental-illness. Last Accessed 30 Sept 2022
3. Mental Health Atlas 2014, In: WHO Library, ISBN 978 92 4 156501 1
4. American Psychological Association. A Summary of Psychologist Workforce Projections: Addressing Supply and Demand from 2015–2030. Washington, DC (2018)
5. Mitchell, A.J, Vaze, A, Rao, S.: Clinical diagnosis of depression in primary care: a meta-analysis. Lancet., 374(9690), 609–19(2009). https://doi.org/10.1016/S0140-6736(09)60879-5. Epub. PMID: 19640579
6. Snowden, L. R.: Bias in mental health assessment and intervention: theory and evidence. Am. J. Public Health 93, 239–243(1993). https://doi.org/10.2105/AJPH.93.2.239
7. Baumel, A., Muench, F., Edan, S., Kane, J.M.: Objective user engagement with mental health apps: systematic search and panel-based usage analysis. J Med Internet Res. **21**(9), e14567 (2019). https://doi.org/10.2196/14567.PMID:31573916;PMCID:PMC6785720.(2019)
8. Muñoz, R.F., Beardslee, W.R., Leykin, Y.: Major depression can be prevented. Am Psychol., 67(4), 285–295(2012). https://doi.org/10.1037/a0027666. PMID: 22583342; PMCID: PMC4533896
9. Thornicroft, G.: Stigma and discrimination limit access to mental health care. Epidemiol Psichiatr Soc. 17(1), 14–9 (2008). https://doi.org/10.1017/s1121189x00002621. PMID: 18444452
10. The Health Insurance Portability and Accountability Act of 1996. Pub. L. 104–191. Stat. 1936. Web. 11 Aug. 2014. (2014)
11. Regulation on the protection of natural persons with regard to the processing of personal data and on the free movement of such data, and repealing Directive 95/46/EC (Data Protection Directive). European Parliament and Council of the European Union, L119, pp. 1–88 (2016)
12. Martinez-Martin, N., Dasgupta, I., Carter, A., Chandler, J., Kellmeyer, P., Kreitmair, K., Weiss, A., Cabrera, L.: Ethics of digital mental health during COVID-19: Crisis and Opportunities. JMIR Ment. Health., 7(12), e23776(2020). https://mental.jmir.org/2020/12/e23776. https://doi.org/10.2196/23776
13. Feijt, M. A., de Kort, Y. A., Bongers, I. M., & IJsselsteijn, W. A.: Perceived drivers and barriers to the adoption of emental health by psychologists: The construction of the levels of adoption of emental health model. J. Med. Internet Res., 20(4), e153(2018). https://doi.org/10.2196/jmir.9485

14. Deshpande, G., Viraraghavan, V.S., Duggirala, M., Reddy, V.R., Patel, S.: Empirical evaluation of emotion classification accuracy for non-acted speech. In: 2017 IEEE 19th International workshop on multimedia signal processing (MMSP) (pp. 1–6). IEEE (2017)
15. Deshpande, G., Viraraghavan, V. S., Duggirala, M., Vempada, R. R., Patel, S.: Comparing manual and machine annotations of emotions in non-acted speech. In: 2018 40th Annual international conference of the ieee engineering in medicine and biology society (EMBC) (pp. 4241–4244). IEEE(2018)
16. Adiga, D. T., Bhavsar, M., Palan, U., Patel, S.: Daily Journals: extracting insights for well-being. In: Proceedings of the 14th EAI International conference on pervasive computing technologies for healthcare (pp. 305–315). Association for Computing Machinery, New York, NY, USA(2020). https://doi.org/10.1145/3421937.3421983
17. Cohen, S., Kamarck, T., Mermelstein, R.: A global measure of perceived stress. J. Health Soc. Behav., 385–396(1983)
18. Agrawal, V., Naik, V., Duggirala, M., Athavale, S.: Color Me: A Game based on art therapy for mental health. In: Extended abstracts of the 2020 Annual Symposium on Computer-Human Interaction in Play (pp. 158–162). Association for Computing Machinery, New York, NY, USA (2020)
19. Deshpande, G., Patel, S., Chanda, S., Patil, P., Agrawal, V., Schuller, B.W.: Laughter as a controller in a stress buster game. In: Proceedings of the 14th EAI International conference on pervasive computing technologies for healthcare (pp. 316–324). Association for Computing Machinery, New York, NY, USA, (2020)
20. Agrawal, V., Naik, V., Duggirala, M., Athavale, S.: Calm a mobile based deep breathing game with biofeedback. In: Extended Abstracts of the 2020 Annual symposium on computer-human interaction in play (pp. 153–157) (2020)
21. Sweller, J.: Cognitive load during problem solving: Effects on learning. Cogn. Sci. **12**(2), 257–285 (1988)
22. Atkinson, R. C., Shiffrin, R. M.: Human memory: A proposed system and its control processes. In: Psychology of learning and motivation, vol. 2, (pp. 89–195). Academic Press (1968)
23. Baddeley, A.: Working memory: looking back and looking forward. Nat. Rev. Neurosci. **4**(10), 829–839 (2003)
24. Csikszentmihalyi, M., Csikzentmihaly, M.: Flow: The psychology of optimal experience (Vol. 1990). Harper & Row, New York (1990)
25. Delle Fave, A., Bassi, M.: The quality of experience in adolescents' daily lives: Developmental perspectives. Genet. Soc. Gen. Psychol. Monogr. **126**(3), 347 (2000)
26. Chandler, P., Sweller, J.: Cognitive load theory and the format of instruction. Cogn. Instr. **8**(4), 293–332 (1991)
27. Sweller, J., Van Merrienboer, J.J., Paas, F.G.: Cognitive architecture and instructional design. Educ. Psychol. Rev. **10**(3), 251–296 (1998)
28. Giovanello, K. S., Verfaellie, M.: Memory systems of the brain: a cognitive neuropsychological analysis. In: Seminars in speech and language (Vol. 22, No. 02, pp. 109–118). Copyright© 2001 by Thieme Medical Publishers, Inc., 333 Seventh Avenue, New York, NY 10001, USA. Tel.:+ 1 (212) 584–4662 (2001)
29. Schifferstein, H.N., Smeets, M.A., Postma, A.: Comparing location memory for 4 sensory modalities. Chem. Senses **35**(2), 135–145 (2010)
30. Csikszentmihalyi, M., Csikszentmihalyi, I. S. (Eds.).: Optimal experience: Psychological studies of flow in consciousness. Cambridge university press (1992)
31. Sinha, A., Gavas, R., Chatterjee, D., Das, R., Sinharay, A.: Dynamic assessment of learners' mental state for an improved learning experience. In: 2015 IEEE frontiers in education conference (FIE) pp. 1–9. IEEE (2015)
32. Morrison, R.E.: Manipulation of stimulus onset delay in reading: evidence for parallel programming of saccades. J. Exp. Psychol. Hum. Percept. Perform. **10**(5), 667 (1984)
33. Hahn, M., Keller, F.: Modeling human reading with neural attention. (2016). arXiv preprint arXiv:1608.05604

34. Deubel, H., O'Regan, K., Radach, R.: Attention, information processing and eye movement control. Read. Percept. Process., 355–374 (2000)
35. Coelli, S., Sclocco, R., Barbieri, R., Reni, G., Zucca, C., Bianchi, A. M.: EEG-based index for engagement level monitoring during sustained attention. In: 2015 37th Annual international conference of the IEEE engineering in medicine and biology society (EMBC) (pp. 1512–1515). IEEE (2015)
36. Schmitt, M., Postma, A., De Haan, E.: Interactions between exogenous auditory and visual spatial attention. Q. J. Exp. Psychol. Sect. A **53**(1), 105–130 (2000)
37. Posner, M.I.: Orienting of attention. Q. J. Exp. Psychol. **32**(1), 3–25 (1980)
38. Posner, M.I., Cohen, Y.: Components of visual orienting. Attention and performance X: Control of language processes **32**, 531–556 (1984)
39. Rayner, K., Well, A.D., Pollatsek, A.: Asymmetry of the effective visual field in reading. Percept. Psychophys. **27**(6), 537–544 (1980)
40. McConkie, G.W., Rayner, K.: The span of the effective stimulus during a fixation in reading. Percept. Psychophys. **17**(6), 578–586 (1975)
41. Jaiswal, D., Chowdhury, A., Banerjee, T., Chatterjee, D.: Effect of mental workload on breathing pattern and heart rate for a working memory task: A pilot study. In: 2019 41st Annual International Conference of the IEEE Engineering in medicine and biology society (EMBC) (pp. 2202–2206). IEEE (2019)
42. Rakshit, R., Reddy, V. R., Deshpande, P.: Emotion detection and recognition using HRV features derived from photoplethysmogram signals. In: Proceedings of the 2nd workshop on emotion representations and modelling for companion systems (pp. 1–6), (2016)
43. Das, P., Chatterjee, D., Ghose, A., Sinha, A.: A system for remote monitoring of mental effort. In: 2016 IEEE 6th International conference on consumer electronics-Berlin (ICCE-Berlin) (pp. 222–226). IEEE (2016)
44. Jackson, S.A., Marsh, H.W.: Development and validation of a scale to measure optimal experience: The flow state scale. J. Sport Exerc. Psychol. **18**(1), 17–35 (1996)
45. Ferstl, E.C., Rinck, M., Cramon, D.Y.V.: Emotional and temporal aspects of situation model processing during text comprehension: An event-related fMRI study. J. Cogn. Neurosci. **17**(5), 724–739 (2005)
46. Hirshfield, L. M., Solovey, E. T., Girouard, A., Kebinger, J., Jacob, R. J., Sassaroli, A., Fantini, S.: Brain measurement for usability testing and adaptive interfaces: an example of uncovering syntactic workload with functional near infrared spectroscopy. In: Proceedings of the SIGCHI Conference on human factors in computing systems (pp. 2185–2194), (2009)
47. Vidaurre, C., Krämer, N., Blankertz, B., Schlögl, A.: Time domain parameters as a feature for EEG-based brain–computer interfaces. Neural. Netw. **22**(9), 1313–1319 (2009)
48. Gavas, R., Chatterjee, D., Sinha, A.: Estimation of cognitive load based on the pupil size dilation. In: 2017 IEEE international conference on systems, man, and cybernetics (SMC) (pp. 1499–1504). IEEE (2017)
49. Singh, N., Aggarwal, Y., Sinha, R.K.: Heart rate variability analysis under varied task difficulties in mental arithmetic performance. Heal. Technol. **9**(3), 343–353 (2019)
50. Serrano, J. P. D., Soltez, J. M. A., Pascual, R. K. C., Castillo, J. C. D., Torres, J. L., Cruz, F. R. G.: Portable stress level detector based on galvanic skin response, heart rate, and body temperature. In: 2018 IEEE 10th International conference on humanoid, nanotechnology, information technology, communication and control, environment and management (HNICEM) (pp. 1–5). IEEE (2018)
51. Chandel, V., Sinharay, A., Ahmed, N., Ghose, A.: Exploiting IMU sensors for IoT enabled health monitoring. In: Proceedings of the First Workshop on IoT-enabled healthcare and wellness technologies and systems (pp. 21–22), (2016)
52. Ahmed, N., Bhattacharyya, C., Ghose, A.: A novel non-parametric approach of tremor detection using wrist-based photoplethysmograph. In: 2020 28th European signal processing conference (EUSIPCO) (pp. 1150–1154). IEEE (2021)
53. Chandel, V., Mukhopadhyay, S., Jaiswal, D., Jani, DS., Khandelwal, S., Pal, A.: C2p: An unobtrusive smartwatch-based platform for automatic background monitoring of fatigue. In:

Proceedings of the first international workshop on human-centered sensing, networking, and systems, (pp. 19–24), (2017)
54. Ahmed, N., Singhal, S., Sharma, V., Bhattacharya, S., Sinha, A., Ghose, A.: A patient-invariant model for freezing of gait detection aided by wavelet decomposition. In: ICASSP 2021–2021 IEEE International conference on acoustics, speech and signal processing (ICASSP) (pp. 1015–1019). IEEE (2021)
55. Gavas, R.D., Chatterjee, D., Sinha, A.: U.S. Patent No. 11,141,061. U.S. Patent and Trademark Office, Washington, DC (2021)
56. Pramanik, H. S., Pal, A., Kirtania, M., Chakravarty, T., Ghose, A.: Smartphone-based sensors in health and wellness monitoring–Perspectives and assessment of the emerging future. In: Smartphone-Based Detection Devices (pp. 375–398). Elsevier (2021)
57. Krishnan, B., Raghavan, V., Vijayakumar, A., Muralidharan, K., Ghose, A., Duggirala, M.: U.S. Patent Application No. 17/199,562 (2021)

# Design Considerations of Mobile Applications for Healthy Living

**Mustafa Degerli**

## 1 Introduction

Mobile health applications, mobile applications specifically designed and developed for health-related purposes, have become more popular, promising, and pervasive in recent years. Additionally, mobile health practices have dependable possibilities to accomplish and improve a comprehensive healthcare system [1]. The use of mobile applications to promote and foster physical activity and activeness was proved to be working [2]. This working scheme needs to be improved with the inputs from relevant stakeholders. It has been verified that mobile applications significantly help to alter several behaviors [3]. A number of notable studies [4] concluded that mobile health applications are truly instrumental to ensure expected changes in behaviors and attain relevant health benefits. Furthermore, users of such apps are generally happy with the use of the relevant apps. For the relevant product and service developers and people using these tools, this is fairly good news.

There are numerous mobile health applications with different maturities available in relevant markets. The mobile application arena is a field where multi and trans-disciplinary efforts are essential for noteworthy success. In addition to the computer science field, business, medicine, economics, and sociology fields ought to be benefited to attain relevant objectives and goals [5]. When relevant cooperation and collaboration are achieved with vigorous involvements in these fields, notable opportunities and improvements are reasonably expected.

Mobile health applications should not be seen as only tools, but they should be designed and developed as prevention strategies. While evaluating these, instead of tool capabilities, actual benefits ought to be analyzed and assessed [6]. Once these instances are distilled and analyzed, both product developers and users are going

M. Degerli (✉)
Graduate School of Informatics, Middle East Technical University, 06800 Ankara, Turkey
e-mail: mustafa.degerli@metu.edu.tr

 
S. Scataglini et al. (eds.), *mHealth and Human-Centered Design Towards Enhanced Health, Care, and Well-Being*, Studies in Big Data 120,
https://doi.org/10.1007/978-981-99-3989-3_6

to feel more confident regarding the use of these apps. Widespread mobile device usage is an important opportunity for underdeveloped and developing countries for sharing health-related information [7]. As these tools are effective means for data and information dissemination and sharing, a significant advantage can be achieved by means of these devices.

In general, the benefits of mobile health applications are encouraging. Nevertheless, individual-level characteristics might create variances in app usage and pertinent perceptions [8]. Therefore, in addition to generic concerns, private and specific expectations or dynamics should be analyzed and implemented in order to ensure a comprehensive accomplishment. In a notable effort [9], usability guidelines for mobile health applications are identified and disseminated. Relevant guidelines highlighted numerous usability items with respect to devoted visual design, refined readability and understandability, improved navigation, delicate feedback, clear notifications, comprehensive help resources and easy troubleshooting, accessible historical data, ensured accessibility, and continuous application evaluation. This type of effort is vital to help developers and end-users for providing or enjoying better experiences.

Naturally, there are different types of mobile health applications in accordance with pertinent use cases, established technical modalities, and relevant applicable policies [10]. This circumstance generates both opportunities and challenges for product developers, marketers, and managers. In this context, smartphones and tablets are more than technological tools in medical and healthcare settings [11]. The apps and hardware of these devices bring about many great opportunities for healthcare delivery professionals and people who want to get healthcare services. This reality creates notable opportunities for end-users, app developers, and even policymakers. In one another study [12], it was reported that people are happy with the improved communication via mobile health applications. In the context of relationship-centered healthcare, mobile health apps are really influential. However, there is a need to better understand the preferences of users and potential users regarding mobile health applications [13]. Further research is expected and required for this context.

The following divisions of this chapter comprise materials about mobile health applications for various situations (Sect. 2) and the important issues related to mobile health applications (Sect. 3). Moreover, the specifics of the research to define design considerations for mobile health applications (Sect. 4) and the identified aspects along with applicable dimensions (Sect. 5) are detailed in the consequent segments. The chapter finalizes with the related discussion (Sect. 6) and conclusions (Sect. 7).

## 2 Mobile Health Applications for Different Purposes

There is a wide spectrum of mobile health applications. Healthy people want to continue their routines with these apps. Moreover, people with chronic diseases and normal people looking for relevant information are all interested in mobile health applications [14]. Mobile health applications are also developed for specific settings. Another main use of mobile health applications can be in workplaces. Promoting health via such apps is a good opportunity. In this manner, the contextual elements of organizations shall not be ignored [15]. Once relevant special dynamics are taken into consideration, the expected benefits are to be notably enhanced. For example, there is a special app developed for office workers to let them work in a healthier manner [16]. Moreover, especially in workplace settings, health promotion leadership can also play a critical role to promote the use of apps [17]. Product managers or policymakers may consider these points for relevant settings.

The recent COVID-19 pandemic that affected the whole world also led to improvements regarding mobile health applications. For example, researchers [18] developed a specific app to address the development of healthy habits via mobile apps. There are also efforts to make use of mobile health applications to help people in rural settings [19]. These works are important so as to increase the coverage of mobile health app users. Oncology is another vital area where several mobile health applications are utilized by healthcare stakeholders (doctors, nurses, patients, etc.) [20]. Such interventions particularly help stakeholders in the oncology domain to facilitate the processes and improve the satisfaction of all stakeholders. Specific mobile health apps for the specific needs of some health professionals, like nurses, are being developed [21]. Such efforts are meaningful as they resolutely address the specific needs and expectations of relevant groups. One other practice space of mobile health applications is multiple sclerosis disease management cases [22]. Providing such apps to people with multiple sclerosis disease provides notably enhanced probabilities for them to administer their health.

Thanks to the ubiquity and accessibility of mobile devices, healthy living and aging can be fairly possible. For example, there are notable works [23] regarding mobile health applications for people with mental illnesses. These people make use of mobile devices and relevant applications to attain and sustain their healthy living and aging. In addition to physical health instances, there are mobile health applications for mental health settings [24], and these apps make use of persuasive design elements.

Still another important promise of mobile health applications is valid and meaningful for older people (seniors) [25]. Older people and their near relatives can benefit from these applications [26] to achieve and maintain their health. Active and healthy living and aging can be supported through these applications. Older people can benefit from these apps to manage and even improve their health. However, from the views of older adults, there are two main points to be improved to ensure the success of mobile health applications [27]. The former problem is that there needs to be a more integrated solution between real-life health services and relevant apps. The latter issue is that cultural and age-related particulars should not be ignored. Taking into consideration the particulars of relevant groups is to enhance the acceptance, adoption, and success of pertinent incentives.

Fundamentally, mobile health applications and wearable medical devices are moderately interrelated. In one work [28], the salience of compatibility, functionality (usability), and motivation (promotion) were verified for wearable medical devices. It is also reasonable to expect that these constructs can also be helpful concerning mobile health applications. It was verified that [29] mobile applications act as motivational influencers for college-age people for a variety of purposes, such as communication, entertainment, education, and other aims. As these recent generations care about respective influencers, this reality and possibility must be taken into account.

Emergency cases are another imperative venue where a significant amount of mobile health applications are developed and available in the relevant markets [30]. As long as the effectiveness and efficiency of these applications are ensured, it will be possible for end-users and caregivers to benefit from these apps in emergency settings. Furthermore, women's pregnancy management domain is still another area where mobile health apps can play critical roles [31]. Nonetheless, more comprehensive and functional apps developed and tested both in developed and developing countries are expected. The related possible evidence shall be studied, tested, and disseminated in these pertinent contexts. Besides, in another interesting work [32], the benefits of using a mobile app by pregnant people were distilled and discussed. Relevant scholars noted the tangible benefits achieved in this situation.

Depression management is another noticeable area, in which a successful mobile health app is developed [33] through a user-centered design methodology. Owing to increased stress and dissatisfaction levels of some people, the use of apps for depression management may be of assistance for pertinent people. Moreover, scholars [34] developed a novel app to improve communication and quality via a rule-based system. Owing to this improvement, the dependability of relevant systems was enhanced. In a notable study [35], researchers developed a service-oriented architecture-based solution to decrease Internet dependency and network infrastructure constraints.

In a remarkable study [36], gamification was incorporated into a mobile app to foster children aged 7–11 and promising results were achieved. As an instance of motivation or persuasion elements, gamification implementations may be helpful for a number of user groups of mobile health applications. People with diabetes also benefit from mobile health applications, and the usability engineering method is a good one to evaluate these specific apps [37]. One other example [38] of the use of mobile apps for health-related purposes regarding a chronic disease, namely asthma, is developed and evaluated. This application has promising potential to help people manage their illnesses and improve their health conditions. There is another notable effort [39] regarding the use of mobile apps for chronic disease prevention and management. As long as the effectiveness of such apps is validated, there is a promising future thanks to the relevant development efforts.

As elaborated and discussed in this part of the chapter, there are numerous efforts and opportunities for product developers and users in the mobile health applications field. Provided that all stakeholders in the relevant settings effectively and efficiently cooperate and collaborate, there is an encouraging future. However, to attain and sustain relevant benefits to the best extent possible, there are some prominent issues to be worked on. The next part of the chapter investigates and examines these components.

## 3 Important Issues About Mobile Health Applications

Fortunately, the Food and Drug Administration of the United States of America issued the first guidance in 2011 on the regulation of mobile medical applications [40]. In this context, it should be noted that there needs to be an equilibrium attained between innovativeness and safety regulations. Too much emphasis on procedures and regulations might hinder relevant developments, and too limited principles may generate undependable products and services.

Privacy of mobile health applications is vital, and there are efforts to fairly address this issue in real applications [41]. Although there are promising developments and useful mobile health apps, the security and privacy of these apps still need significant improvements [42]. In a study [43], significant privacy deficiencies of mobile health applications have been reviewed and deliberated. This issue needs to be fixed to both comply with the relevant regulations and ensure people's trust. There is a good example of the design and development of a mobile health application [44] that satisfies both security and privacy expectations. Although it is quite a few, seeing such successful interventions is promising for the present and future of mobile health applications. Privacy issues need solutions when many current mobile health applications are considered [45]. This reality should be taken into account by both developers and users. Unless these components are also adequately addressed, the expected benefits are to be remarkably jeopardized.

Identifying and addressing the views and expectations of users and clinicians are going to be beneficial for the success of mobile applications [46]. Since these actors have significant information and experience regarding the pertinent practices and success, their contributions are remarkably and positively going to influence the processes and products. Developers of mobile health applications should consider the mobile device characteristics of different users. That is, it should not be overlooked that some people may have low-end devices and they also want to get benefit from the advantages provided with the pertinent apps. To address this concern, lightweight and/or cloud-based solutions may also be incorporated [47]. It is also legitimate to design and develop hybrid (mobile health cloud app with a native container) mobile health apps to merge the advantages of mobile native apps and cloud mobile apps [48]. This kind of opportunity is to increase the coverage and realized the benefits of applicable applications.

Verification and validation activities in order to ensure the dependability of the subject mobile health applications are extremely imperative owing to the fact that these apps may affect people's health [49]. Doing the right thing right in these contexts is going to provide confidence to all people involved. Validation of mobile health applications is expected and required. Furthermore, management issues, usability concerns, ethics views, and network realities [50] are some of the main drivers regarding mobile health applications. As long as these drivers are addressed and managed, the success of relevant incentives can be notably sustained and enhanced.

As long as good design, quality of information, competent people, and compatibility constructs are ensured, there is a high potential for people with dementia to benefit from mobile health applications to manage and improve their social, physical, and mental health dynamics [51]. Although the importance of these factors is verified for these special groups and apps, the salience of these items can also be evaluated as valid and worthy for different groups and most of the mobile health applications. Besides, customization options and design elements are important to be considered during the development of mobile health applications to realize user-centered solutions [52]. Such efforts are going to particularly lead to the success of relevant apps regarding the views of users. In addition to functionality, people care about aesthetics and personalization, and this should not be missed by product developers or managers. The design and usability of mobile health applications are firmly shaping the user satisfaction and loyalty. In this context, the involvements of relevant people in the design stages are crucial [53]. This kind of implementation is to provide low-cost fixations and improvements since relevant feedback is gotten and incorporated before it is too late and costly.

The quality of mobile health applications is imperative as these may sometimes be life-threatening. Safety, security, privacy, usability, interoperability, learnability, reliability, and portability are major quality factors for mobile health applications [54]. All these quality factors must be given the required importance to produce and maintain dependable products. A variety of technical optimization tools like fuzzy optimization can be used to enhance systems regarding mobile health settings [55]. These technical and engineering works are going to improve the effectiveness and efficiency of relevant works. Furthermore, the model decision, data management, and trade-offs are the main issues for optimizations of mobile health interventions. For example, in a work [56], reinforcement learning as a branch of machine learning was used to optimize behavioral health. Applying these popular engineering applications also provides improvement opportunities.

Unfortunately, scientific evaluation and expert involvement are two mostly ignored factors in mobile health applications aimed at weight management of people [57]. This sort of ignorance brings about major problems regarding the dependability of relevant products. For sustainable development, mobile health applications should also take location information and contexts into consideration [58]. Such kind of an implementation expands the experience and usage of relevant apps. Moreover, persuasive mobile apps for health purposes are beneficial to help people attain and sustain healthy lifestyles [59]. People sometimes expect and like different kinds of incentives or motivators to start or go further.

The usability of mobile health applications must be supported with safety, security, and interoperability constructs [60]. Obviously, functions are important. Yet, unless these are accompanied by these important facets, the relevant success is to be negatively affected. Besides, aesthetic design, functionality, and usability are the three focal design issues for mobile applications [61], and this domain needs improvements to better understand and manage relevant settings. Dialogue support and social support functions along with rewards and networking features are generally missing when most breastfeeding mobile health applications are evaluated [62]. As long as these functions and features are incorporated, acceptance, adoption, and success of relevant apps may be enhanced. By the way, in addition to breastfeeding mobile health apps, these features can also be favorable for a variety of mobile health applications.

People's quality perception, customization opportunities in accordance with people's preferences, and associated potential threats are noted as the main elements for the adoption of mobile health applications [63]. Product developers ought to consider all these in related design and development works. The utilization of collected data through mobile health applications should be improved among users and healthcare professionals [64]. The collection of relevant data can only be fully meaningful as long as these are meaningfully used. Additionally, in a study [65], the possible impact of word of mouth, health awareness, and disease threat perception was distilled and discussed concerning mobile health applications. Moreover, determining potential customers and defining the values to be delivered are the main topics that should be addressed by the mobile health start-up organizations first before going further regarding product or service development and provision [66] as these are to enhance their potential success.

The dependability (reliability and quality) of mobile health applications for older people needs more examination and analysis [67]. The outcomes of these analyses must be scientifically derived and systematically discussed. Trust is an important element of mobile health application success [68]. People should feel confident regarding the benefits and reliability of pertinent apps. In addition to basic factors of the unified theory of acceptance and use of technology, cognitive trust and ratings were determined to be leading for healthcare professionals regarding mobile health apps [69]. Therefore, product developers and managers outgo to take measures to establish cognitive trust and actively monitor evaluations.

In a study [70], for a special mobile healthcare system, the importance of ease of use was explored and verified. It is not enough to be only useful for apps, relevant apps should also be easy to use for the expected acceptance and adoption of these interventions. More personal and customizable mobile health applications along with interactive feedback mechanisms are expected by people for healthy living conditions [71]. Besides, assistive and persuasive mobile health applications can help people attain and sustain their objectives and goals [72]. For example, people at the college level prefer visually refined, customizable, and not-competitive apps, when they evaluate a specific mobile health application [73]. This also notably highlights the importance of design elements concerning mobile health applications. When people see tangible benefits along with motivational items, it is easier for them to advance. Hence, product developers and managers must be aware of this reality too.

Designers and developers of mobile health applications need to be trained to let them ensure better performance regarding their product's privacy, usability, and security components [74]. Additionally, human factor optimization is fairly important for mobile health applications, which help to democratize health accessibility especially in developing regions of the world [75]. Besides, sound risk management practices should be followed and implemented to ensure that associated possible threats do not harm people's health thru mobile medical applications [76]. In one study [77], it was determined that there is a need to develop evidence-based and theory-driven mobile health apps for mental health management. The effectiveness of apps should be verified and validated thru comprehensive scientific scenarios. Furthermore, for older people, the cases of mobile health interventions should be designed and implemented with the contribution of all relevant stakeholders [78]. End-users, experts, and family members may help with their views and experiences.

There are different attempts to evaluate people's satisfaction with the mobile health apps they use. For instance, scholars [79] developed a questionnaire for this purpose and used that for an app. The quality and quantity of these tools should be increased as these are guiding for users and developers. There is still a need for an evaluation framework to be used by end-users to evaluate the quality and usability of mobile health applications [80]. Additionally, tools and platforms to evaluate mobile health and medical apps still need improvements to both guide developers and let users evaluate relevant apps [81]. Once such scales are drafted and refined, people may have better chances and knowledge to decide on the use. Additionally, the effectiveness of applications and design of applications were determined [82] to be two main areas that are open for improvements regarding mobile health applications related to obesity management.

Besides, taking measures to ensure the motivation and engagement of people towards relevant mobile health apps is recommended to increase the effectiveness of treatments through the pertinent apps [83]. In one analysis [84], the importance of benefits, and functionalities, was verified for the acceptance of mobile health applications. Moreover, qualities of information, service, and design leading to intimacy are three major forces for mobile apps to succeed [85]. Additionally, there are six main design considerations planned and implemented for a health service platform. These are adaptability, accessibility, interoperability, evolvability, flexibility, and reusability [86]. Such facets can also be meaningful for mobile health applications since they are fundamentally interdepended to a certain extent.

All these details prove that there are rooms for improvements concerning mobile health applications. Unambiguously, understanding people's views and expectations better on the subject of design considerations of mobile applications for healthy living can help product developers and policymakers. That's why this devoted research work was conducted for this purpose, and details and results of the relevant work are shared in the following parts of this chapter to modestly add to the pertinent body of knowledge and experience.

## 4 Research Design and Elements

With the intention of investigating and distilling relevant design consideration themes and pertinent items, a two-part survey was drafted and conducted in the subject research. The first part of the instrument included demographical questions, and the second part included some statements to get participants' views concerning how they rate the statements thru a Likert-type scale (from 1 to 5).

The reliability of the instrument was evaluated based on Cronbach's alpha value and 0.88 was calculated, positively exceeding the relevant threshold (~0.70). Moreover, two experts provided reviews and inputs to confirm and improve the content validity of the instrument.

After ensuring the reliability and validity of the questionnaire, pertinent data were collected from 245 people from Turkey by means of the survey. Specifically, convenience sampling is applied in this context. Questionnaires were distributed online. Before starting the survey, each participant's informed consent was guaranteed. Participants were allowed to stop and quit the work whenever they want to do so.

Frequency details of the collected data regarding the participants are given in Tables 1 and 2. Relevant particulars in the given tables show that the collected data are moderately comprehensive and representative to make legitimately generalizable conclusions.

In order to explore and confirm relevant relations with respect to data collected, by using IBM's SPSS package, the exploratory factor analysis method was followed and applied. Owing to that the pertinent data were collected from 245 different people, the method's relevant size requirement (N > 200) was sufficiently met. During following the relevant analysis approach, the anti-image correlation matrix was created and investigated to ensure factorability. Besides, requirements for sample size tests (Kaiser-Meier-Olkin—KMO and Bartlett's) were satisfied and values for commonalities extracted were analyzed to ensure full conformance to the method

**Table 1** Frequency details of the participants

| *Gender* | N | % |
|---|---|---|
| Women | 119 | 48.57 |
| Men | 126 | 51.43 |
| *Age* | | |
| 16–24 | 27 | 11.02 |
| 25–34 | 95 | 38.78 |
| 35–54 | 79 | 32.24 |
| 55+ | 44 | 17.96 |
| *Education* | | |
| Primary School | 9 | 3.67 |
| Secondary School | 17 | 6.94 |
| B.Sc. | 160 | 65.31 |
| M.Sc. | 45 | 18.37 |
| Ph.D. | 14 | 5.71 |
| *Income* | | |
| Low | 35 | 14.29 |
| Mid | 141 | 57.55 |
| High | 69 | 28.16 |

**Table 2** Frequency details of the participants concerning mobile app and mobile health app usage

| *Mobile app users* | N | % |
|---|---|---|
| Yes | 223 | 91.02 |
| No | 22 | 8.98 |
| *Mobile health app users* | | |
| Yess | 138 | 56.33 |
| No | 107 | 43.67 |

requirements. Accordingly, three themes with 13 instances were investigated and established. The total variance explained was 77.36%.

## 5 Design Considerations of Mobile Health Applications

Applied exploratory factor analysis concluded that there are three aspects and 13 relevant items regarding the design considerations of mobile applications for healthy living. Table 3 reflects the definitions and relevant items for the applicable design considerations.

**Table 3** Design considerations for mobile health applications

| Compatibility (C)<br>*Applications need to comply with the routines and behaviors of people using* | |
|---|---|
| C1 | Work with ordinary smartphones |
| C2 | Work with wearable smartwatches |
| C3 | Behavior modifications are gradually realized |
| C4 | Users are not significantly disturbed |
| Functionality (F)<br>*Applications ought to provide distinct benefits to people using* | |
| F1 | Show how the users perform with respect to requirements |
| F2 | Show how the app helps the users to reach their health-related objectives |
| F3 | Include interactive help capabilities |
| F4 | Ensure the expected benefits |
| F5 | Meet the users' exact needs |
| Motivation (M)<br>*Applications must encourage people to use them* | |
| M1 | Push customizable notifications and reminders |
| M2 | Include gamification features |
| M3 | Award tags or badges for the continuous performance |
| M4 | Provide tips to meet the requirements |

With respect to their relevant weights, the three main considerations can be listed, from the highest to the lowest, as functionality, compatibility, and motivation. Namely, the first thing people look for is the functionality. People expect distinct benefits from the relevant mobile health applications. After the functionality, people prioritize the compatibility facet. Users look for relevant apps that comply with their routines and behaviors. In addition to functionality and compatibility, people give importance to the motivation component. Individuals await some kind of encouragement to use the relevant mobile health applications.

13 crucial features under these three central topics given in Table 3 were distilled with respect to people's views and expectations, which mostly govern the success of mobile health applications. Table 3 can be used by product developers and people making pertinent policies to improve the products and/or policies. The items and themes can be used entirely or partially, as applicable, by the interested parties concerning their priorities or available resources.

## 6 Discussion

As long as designed and used appropriately, mobile health practices and mobile health applications can actually be beneficial and instrumental to attain and improve the health and well-being of most people [1]. Both healthy people and people with illnesses can benefit from mobile health applications [14]. As long as all participants in mobile health application venues cooperate and collaborate successfully and competently, there are great opportunities and progressive outlooks for all relevant stakeholders.

Privacy and security issues of mobile health applications still need more dedicated studies, investigations, and efforts [41]–[45]. As these two issues are to govern people's trust and confidence, product developers and policymakers need to appreciate the importance and relevant requirements. Addressing only engineering works will not be enough to deliver fully successful solutions.

There is a need to better understand people's views and comments on mobile health applications [13]. The subject research detailed in this chapter tried to answer further research calls in this context. As also confirmed in the scope of the subject research detailed in this chapter, usability, compatibility, user views, motivational elements, and customizability are important features for the accomplishment of mobile health applications [14, 46, 50, 52, 53, 63, 72, 84].

Designing, developing, and publishing a mobile health application meeting the requirements of functionality, compatibility, and motivation themes are going to be wise steps for relevant stakeholders. In this context, specifically, applications should provide distinct benefits to people using, must comply with the routines and behaviors of people using, and ought to encourage people to use these apps. As long as these design considerations are understood and addressed, the full potential of mobile health applications can be realized and perfected. For this purpose, the checklist included in Table 3 in Sect. 5 of this chapter can be utilized by relevant stakeholders.

Obviously, functionality, compatibility, and motivation constructs are not the only design considerations that guarantee the expected accomplishment. Further efforts are still required to distill other design considerations of mobile health applications. Unambiguously, convenience, promotions, and quality aspects along with relevant items can be studied and discussed in further investigations.

Evaluations and even certifications of mobile health applications with respect to comprehensive design considerations criteria by authorized and dependable organizations might also be a good idea. This kind of effort might be going to provide confidence to both developers and users regarding the pertinent mobile health applications. Such kind of mechanism might be optional and organizations may want to be part of this to ensure the quality and dependability.

Especially in cases of developing countries, mobile health applications can be classified by relevant authorities, and for the required categories of relevant applications, rigorous review, evaluation, and approval processes can be put into practice to ensure that health-related apps are satisfactorily qualified and dependable.

## 7 Conclusions

Through doing a literature review and analysis, this chapter included particulars concerning mobile health applications for various purposes. Besides, a discussion on important issues regarding mobile health applications was incorporated. Furthermore, this chapter provided details about the originally particularized and examined design considerations of mobile health applications. In this context, 13 crucial features for three principal themes were given. Product developers and managers in the context of the mobile health applications field may benefit from this chapter to evaluate their products and services and can identify some opportunities for improvement. Policymakers might have a look at this chapter to better understand the mobile health applications field and gain insights to draft or refine relevant policies. Other scholars can use this chapter to grasp available mobile health applications, current pertinent issues, and meaningful design considerations to take as inputs for their scientific efforts. The present and future of the mobile health applications field are bright, and further engineering and interdisciplinary works are required and expected in order to realize the full potential of mobile health applications for all pertinent stakeholders.

## References

1. Vasudevan, L., Zeller, K., Labrique, A.: Mobile Health. In: Rivas, H., Wac, K. (Eds.) Digital health, health informatics, pp. 15–25. Springer International Publishing AG 2018 (2018). https://doi.org/10.1007/978-3-319-61446-5_2

2. Muntaner, A., Vidal-Conti, J., Palou, P.: Increasing physical activity through mobile device interventions: A systematic review. Health Informatics J. **22**(3), 451–469 (2016). https://doi.org/10.1177/1460458214567004
3. Paula, T. R., de Menezes, A. P., Guedes, N. G., da Silva, V. M., Cardoso, M. V. L. M. L., de S. Ramos, E. S.: Effectiveness of mobile applications for behavioral changes in health: a systematic review. Rev Rene, **21**, e43845 (2020). https://doi.org/10.15253/2175-6783.20202143845
4. Han, M., Lee, E.: Effectiveness of mobile health application use to improve health behavior changes: a systematic review of randomized controlled trials. Healthcare Informatics Research **24**(3), 207 (2018). https://doi.org/10.4258/hir.2018.24.3.207
5. Degerli, M.: An overview of mobile health applications and development of an original mobile health application. EMO Sci. J, **11**(21), 59–69 (2021). [Online]. https://dergipark.org.tr/tr/pub/emobd/issue/63506/888041
6. Aromatario, O., et al.: How do mobile health applications support behaviour changes? A scoping review of mobile health applications relating to physical activity and eating behaviours. Public Health **175**, 8–18 (2019). https://doi.org/10.1016/j.puhe.2019.06.011
7. Angula, N., Dlodlo, N.: Mobile technology for health information dissemination. In: 2017 IST-Africa Week Conference (IST-Africa) (pp. 1–8), (2017). https://doi.org/10.23919/ISTAFRICA.2017.8102329
8. Bhuyan, S.S., et al.: Use of mobile health applications for health-seeking behavior among us adults. J. Med. Syst. **40**(6), 153 (2016). https://doi.org/10.1007/s10916-016-0492-7
9. Roy, B., Call, M., Abts, N.: Development of usability guidelines for mobile health applications. In: Communications in Computer and Information Science, vol. 1034, (pp. 500–506). Springer Verlag, (2019). https://doi.org/10.1007/978-3-030-23525-3_68
10. Olla, P., Shimskey, C.: mHealth taxonomy: a literature survey of mobile health applications. Heal. Technol. **4**(4), 299–308 (2015). https://doi.org/10.1007/s12553-014-0093-8
11. Agarwal, A., Furht, B., Yenagi, M.: Mobile medical and healthcare applications. In: Furht, B., Agarwal, A (Eds) Handbook of Medical and Healthcare Technologies, pp. 3–15. Springer New York, NY (2013). https://doi.org/10.1007/978-1-4614-8495-0_1.
12. Qudah, B., Luetsch, K.: The influence of mobile health applications on patient—healthcare provider relationships: A systematic, narrative review. Patient Educ. Couns. **102**(6), 1080–1089 (2019). https://doi.org/10.1016/j.pec.2019.01.021
13. Baig, M.M., GholamHosseini, H., Connolly, M.J.: Mobile healthcare applications: system design review, critical issues and challenges. Australas. Phys. Eng. Sci. Med. **38**(1), 23–38 (2015). https://doi.org/10.1007/s13246-014-0315-4
14. García-Gómez, J.M., de la Torre-Díez, I., Vicente, J., Robles, M., López-Coronado, M., Rodrigues, J.J.: Analysis of mobile health applications for a broad spectrum of consumers: A user experience approach. Health Informatics J. **20**(1), 74–84 (2014). https://doi.org/10.1177/1460458213479598
15. Melzner, J., Heinze, J., Fritsch, T.: Mobile health applications in workplace health promotion: an integrated conceptual adoption framework. Procedia Technol. **16**, 1374–1382 (2014). https://doi.org/10.1016/j.protcy.2014.10.155
16. Degerli, M.: A mobile health application for healthy living: HWOW (Healthier Work for Office Workers). In: 2020 Turkish national software engineering symposium (UYMS) (pp. 1–3), (2020). https://doi.org/10.1109/UYMS50627.2020.9247024
17. Bregenzer, A., Wagner-Hartl, V., Jiménez, P.: Who uses apps in health promotion? A target group analysis of leaders. Health Informatics J. **25**(3), 1038–1052 (2019). https://doi.org/10.1177/1460458217738121
18. Palacios-Gálvez, M.S., Andrés-Villas, M., Vélez-Toral, M., Merino-Godoy, Á.: Nominal groups to develop a mobile application on healthy habits. Healthcare **9**(4), 378 (2021). https://doi.org/10.3390/healthcare9040378
19. Larson, K.L., et al.: A contextual approach to inform a mobile health application for adolescent health. J. Child Fam. Stud. **29**(12), 3420–3432 (2020). https://doi.org/10.1007/s10826-020-01826-x

20. Doyle-Lindrud, S.: Mobile health technology and the use of health-related mobile applications. Clin. J. Oncol. Nurs. **18**(6), 634–636 (2014). https://doi.org/10.1188/14.CJON.634-636
21. O'Connor, S., Andrews, T.: Co-designing Mobile apps to assist in clinical nursing education: A study protocol. Stud. Health Technol. Inform. **225**, 963–964 (2016). https://doi.org/10.3233/978-1-61499-658-3-963
22. Giunti, G., Guisado-Fernandez, E., Caulfield, B.: Connected health in multiple sclerosis: a mobile applications review. In: 2017 IEEE 30th International Symposium on Computer-Based Medical Systems (CBMS), vol. 2017-June, (pp. 660–665), (2017). https://doi.org/10.1109/CBMS.2017.27
23. Li, H., Lewis, C., Chi, H., Singleton, G., Williams, N.: Mobile health applications for mental illnesses: An Asian context. Asian J. Psychiatry, **54**(June), 102209(2020). https://doi.org/10.1016/j.ajp.2020.102209
24. Chang, T.-R., Kaasinen, E., Kaipainen, K.: Persuasive design in mobile applications for mental well-being: multidisciplinary expert review. In: lecture notes of the institute for computer sciences. Social-Informatics and Telecommunications Engineering, LNICST **61**, 154–162 (2013). https://doi.org/10.1007/978-3-642-37893-5_18
25. Helbostad, J., et al.: Mobile health applications to promote active and healthy ageing. Sensors **17**(3), 622 (2017). https://doi.org/10.3390/s17030622
26. Li, H.H., Chang, C.T., Liao, Y.-H.: Using mobile application for Long-Term Care system. In: 2015 Eighth International conference on mobile computing and ubiquitous networking (ICMU), (pp. 62–63), (2015). https://doi.org/10.1109/ICMU.2015.7061030
27. Karaca Şalgamcıoğlu, B.: Future older adults and mobile applications for health. In: Design of assistive technology for ageing populations, vol. 167, no. 3001744230, (pp. 275–292), (2020). https://doi.org/10.1007/978-3-030-26292-1_15
28. Degerli, M., Ozkan Yildirim, S.: Identifying critical success factors for wearable medical devices: a comprehensive exploration. Univers. Access Inf. Soc., 21(1), 121–143. https://doi.org/10.1007/s10209-020-00763-2
29. Mutchler, L. A., Shim, J. P.: Mobile Apps : Motivational influencers emergent research forum paper. In: Twenty-third Americas Conference on Information Systems (pp. 1–5). (2017)
30. Plaza Roncero, A. et al.: Mobile health apps for medical emergencies: systematic review. JMIR Mhealth Uhealth, **8**(12), e18513(2020). https://doi.org/10.2196/18513
31. Iyawa, G.E., Dansharif, A.R., Khan, A.: Mobile apps for self-management in pregnancy: a systematic review. Heal. Technol. **11**(2), 283–294 (2021). https://doi.org/10.1007/s12553-021-00523-z
32. Sommer, J., Daus, M., Smith, M., Luna, D.: Mobile application for pregnant women: What do mothers say?. In: MEDINFO 2017: Precision Healthcare through Informatics, vol. 245, (pp. 221–224), (2017). https://doi.org/10.3233/978-1-61499-830-3-221
33. Callan, J.A., et al.: CBT mobilework©: user-centered development and testing of a mobile mental health application for depression. Cogn. Ther. Res. **45**(2), 287–302 (2021). https://doi.org/10.1007/s10608-020-10159-4
34. Rodrigues, N., Vilaça, J. L.: A mobile health care rule-based system. In: Communications in Computer and Information Science, vol. 221 CCIS, no. PART 3, (pp. 371–383), (2011). https://doi.org/10.1007/978-3-642-24352-3_39
35. Silva, B.M.C., Rodrigues, J.J.P.C., Lopes, I.M.C., Machado, T.M.F., Zhou, L.: A novel cooperation strategy for mobile health applications. IEEE J. Sel. Areas Commun. **31**(9), 28–36 (2013). https://doi.org/10.1109/JSAC.2013.SUP.0513003
36. Hill, D. et al.: Mobile technologies for promoting health and wellness among African American Youth. In: Lecture notes in computer science (including subseries lecture notes in artificial intelligence and lecture notes in bioinformatics), vol. 6767 LNCS, no. PART 3, (pp. 36–45). (2011). https://doi.org/10.1007/978-3-642-21666-4_5
37. Georgsson, M.: A review of usability methods used in the evaluation of mobile health applications for diabetes. In pHealth 2020, vol. 273, (pp. 228–233), (2020). https://doi.org/10.3233/SHTI200645

38. Cook, S., Sembajwe, R., Massoudi, B., Recker, A.: An app a day keeps the doctor…informed: user evaluation of a patient mobile health application and clinician dashboard. In: Communications in computer and information science, vol. 374, no. PART II, (pp. 153–157). (2013). https://doi.org/10.1007/978-3-642-39476-8_32
39. Ding, H., Varnfield, M., Karunanithi, M.: Mobile applications towards prevention and management of chronic diseases. In: Lecture notes in computer science (including subseries lecture notes in artificial intelligence and lecture notes in bioinformatics), vol. 7235 LNCS, (pp. 788–791), (2012). https://doi.org/10.1007/978-3-642-29253-8_79
40. Barton, A.J.: The regulation of mobile health applications. BMC Med. **10**(1), 46 (2012). https://doi.org/10.1186/1741-7015-10-46
41. Lin, W., Xu, M., He, J., Zhang, W.: Privacy, security and resilience in mobile healthcare applications. Enterp. Inf. Syst. **00**(00), 1–15 (2021). https://doi.org/10.1080/17517575.2021.1939896
42. Aliasgari, M., Black, M., Yadav, N.: Security vulnerabilities in mobile health applications. In: 2018 IEEE Conference on application, information and network security (AINS) (pp. 21–26). https://doi.org/10.1109/AINS.2018.8631464
43. Papageorgiou, A., Strigkos, M., Politou, E., Alepis, E., Solanas, A., Patsakis, C.: Security and privacy analysis of mobile health applications: the alarming state of practice. IEEE Access **6**, 9390–9403 (2018). https://doi.org/10.1109/ACCESS.2018.2799522
44. Volk, M., Sterle, J., Sedlar, U.: Safety and privacy considerations for mobile application design in digital healthcare. Int. J. Distrib. Sens. Netw. **2015**(1), 1–12 (2015). https://doi.org/10.1155/2015/549420
45. Rowan, M., Dehlinger, J.: A privacy policy comparison of health and fitness related mobile applications. Procedia Comput. Sci. **37**, 348–355 (2014). https://doi.org/10.1016/j.procs.2014.08.051
46. Fahlevi, M.: Mobile applications for health management in Indonesia. In: 2020 International Conference on Information Management and Technology (ICIMTech), no. August, (pp. 324–329). https://doi.org/10.1109/ICIMTech50083.2020.9211243
47. Emamian, P., Li, J.: SimpleHealth—A mobile cloud platform to support lightweight mobile health applications for low-end cellphones. In: 2017 IEEE 19th International Conference on e-Health Networking, Applications and Services (Healthcom), vol. 2017-Decem, (pp. 1–6), (2017). https://doi.org/10.1109/HealthCom.2017.8210759
48. Martinez-Perez, B., de la Torre-Diez, I., Lopez-Coronado, M., Rodrigues, J.J.P.C.: Are mobile health cloud apps better than native? In: 2015 IEEE International Conference on Communications (ICC), vol. 2015-Septe, (pp. 518–523), (2015). https://doi.org/10.1109/ICC.2015.7248374
49. Suman, R., Sahibuddin, S.: User acceptance testing in mobile health applications. In: Proceedings of the 2019 2nd international conference on information science and systems, vol. Part F1483, (pp. 145–149), (2019). https://doi.org/10.1145/3322645.3322670
50. Pires, I.M., Marques, G., Garcia, N.M., Flórez-Revuelta, F., Ponciano, V., Oniani, S.: A research on the classification and applicability of the mobile health applications. J. Pers. Med. **10**(1), 11 (2020). https://doi.org/10.3390/jpm10010011
51. Brown, A., O'Connor, S.: Mobile health applications for people with dementia: a systematic review and synthesis of qualitative studies. Inform. Health Soc. Care **45**(4), 343–359 (2020). https://doi.org/10.1080/17538157.2020.1728536
52. Wang, X., Du, K., Zhu, K., Xu, S., Zhang, S.: Where should mobile health application providers focus their goals? Int. J. Comput. Intell. Syst. **14**(1), 1119 (2021). https://doi.org/10.2991/ijcis.d.210305.001
53. Shah, U., Chiew, T.: A systematic literature review of the design approach and usability evaluation of the pain management mobile applications. Symmetry (Basel) **11**(3), 400 (2019). https://doi.org/10.3390/sym11030400
54. Lechner, N.H., Strahonja, V.: Quality factors for mobile medical apps. Cent.L Eur. Conf. Inf. Intell. Syst. **2014**, 229–236 (2017)

55. Mezei, J., Nikou, S.: Fuzzy optimization to improve mobile health and wellness recommendation systems. Knowl.-Based Syst. **142**, 108–116 (2018). https://doi.org/10.1016/j.knosys.2017.11.030
56. Figueroa, C.A., et al.: Adaptive learning algorithms to optimize mobile applications for behavioral health: guidelines for design decisions. J. Am. Med. Inform. Assoc. **28**(6), 1225–1234 (2021). https://doi.org/10.1093/jamia/ocab001
57. Rivera, J., et al.: Mobile apps for weight management: a scoping review. JMIR Mhealth Uhealth **4**(3), e87 (2016). https://doi.org/10.2196/mhealth.5115
58. Nyapwere, N., Dube, Y.P., Makanga, P.T.: Guidelines for developing geographically sensitive mobile health applications. Heal. Technol. **11**(2), 379–387 (2021). https://doi.org/10.1007/s12553-020-00518-2
59. Garcia Wylie, C., Coulton, P.: Persuasive mobile health applications. In: Electronic Healthcare, vol. 1 LNICST, (pp. 90–97). Springer Berlin Heidelberg, Berlin, Heidelberg, (2009). https://doi.org/10.1007/978-3-642-00413-1_11
60. Jones, J. F., Hook, S. A., Park, S. C., Scott, L. M.: Privacy, security and interoperability of mobile health applications. In: Lecture notes in computer science (including subseries lecture notes in artificial intelligence and lecture notes in bioinformatics), vol. 6767 LNCS, no. PART 3, (pp. 46–55). (2011). https://doi.org/10.1007/978-3-642-21666-4_6
61. Huang, Z., Tian, Z.: Analysis and design for mobile applications: a user experience approach. In: DUXU, LNCS, vol. 10918, (pp. 91–100). Springer International Publishing, (2018). https://doi.org/10.1007/978-3-319-91797-9_7
62. Meedya, S., Sheikh, M.K., Win, K.T., Halcomb, E.: Evaluation of breastfeeding mobile health applications based on the persuasive system design model. In: Lecture notes in computer science (including subseries lecture notes in artificial intelligence and lecture notes in bioinformatics), vol. 11433 LNCS (pp. 189–201). Springer International Publishing, (2019). https://doi.org/10.1007/978-3-030-17287-9_16
63. Saheb, T.: An empirical investigation of the adoption of mobile health applications: integrating big data and social media services. Heal. Technol. **10**(5), 1063–1077 (2020). https://doi.org/10.1007/s12553-020-00422-9
64. Zangger, M., Wälchli, C., Stefenelli, U., Stute, P.: The use of mobile health applications for the prevention of non-communicable diseases. Heal. Technol. **11**(3), 585–593 (2021). https://doi.org/10.1007/s12553-021-00536-8
65. Birkmeyer, S., Wirtz, B. W., Langer, P. F.: Determinants of mHealth success: An empirical investigation of the user perspective. Int. J. Inf. Manag., **59**(March), 102351(2021). https://doi.org/10.1016/j.ijinfomgt.2021.102351
66. Lux, T., Kempf, Y.: Success factors for market entry of mobile health startups. In: 2021 IEEE/ACS 18th International conference on computer systems and applications (AICCSA), 2021-Decem, 1–4(2021). https://doi.org/10.1109/AICCSA53542.2021.9686849
67. Berauk, V.L.A., Murugiah, M.K., Soh, Y.C., Sheng, Y.C., Wong, T.W., Ming, L.C.: Mobile health applications for caring of older people: review and comparison. Ther. Innov. & Regul. Sci. **52**(3), 374–382 (2018). https://doi.org/10.1177/2168479017725556
68. Doğanyiğit, S. Ö.: Exploring intention on continuous use of mobile health applications designed by persuasive technology: 'Adimsayar' case study. In: Current and Emerging mHealth Technologies (pp. 37–53). Springer International Publishing, Cham(2018). https://doi.org/10.1007/978-3-319-73135-3_4.
69. Wu, P., Zhang, R., Luan, J., Zhu, M.: Factors affecting physicians using mobile health applications: an empirical study. BMC Health Serv. Res. **22**(24), 1–14 (2022). https://doi.org/10.1186/s12913-021-07339-7
70. Keikhosrokiani, P., Mustaffa, N., Zakaria, N., Abdullah, R.: Assessment of a medical information system: the mediating role of use and user satisfaction on the success of human interaction with the mobile healthcare system (iHeart). Cogn. Technol. Work **22**(2), 281–305 (2020). https://doi.org/10.1007/s10111-019-00565-4
71. Simons, L.P.A., Hampe, J.F., Guldemond, N.A.: Designing healthy living support: mobile applications added to hybrid (e)Coach solution. Heal. Technol. **3**(1), 85–95 (2013). https://doi.org/10.1007/s12553-013-0052-9

72. Connelly, K. H., Faber, A. M., Rogers, Y., Siek, K. A., Toscos, T.: Mobile applications that empower people to monitor their personal health. E & I Elektrotechnik Und Inf.Stechnik, **123**(4), 124–128(2006). https://doi.org/10.1007/s00502-006-0326
73. Warnick, J.L., Pfammatter, A., Champion, K., Galluzzi, T., Spring, B.: Perceptions of health behaviors and mobile health applications in an academically elite college population to inform a targeted health promotion program. Int. J. Behav. Med. **26**(2), 165–174 (2019). https://doi.org/10.1007/s12529-018-09767-y
74. Asaddok, N., Ghazali, M.: Exploring the usability, security and privacy taxonomy for mobile health applications. In: 2017 International conference on research and innovation in information systems (ICRIIS) (pp. 1–6), (2017). https://doi.org/10.1109/ICRIIS.2017.8002472
75. Schwab, T., Langell, J.: Human Factors-based mobile application design for global health. Surg. Innov. **25**(6), 557–562 (2018). https://doi.org/10.1177/1553350618814643
76. Moshi, M.R., Parsons, J., Tooher, R., Merlin, T.: Evaluation of mobile health applications: is regulatory policy up to the challenge? Int. J. Technol. Assess. Health Care **35**(4), 351–360 (2019). https://doi.org/10.1017/S0266462319000461
77. Hwang, W.J., Ha, J.S., Kim, M.J.: Research trends on mobile mental health application for general population: a scoping review. Int. J. Environ. Res. Public Health **18**(5), 2459 (2021). https://doi.org/10.3390/ijerph18052459
78. Tu, J., Shen, M., Zhong, J., Yuan, G., Chen, M.: The perceptions and experiences of mobile health technology by older people in guangzhou, china: a qualitative study. Front. Public Health **9**(June), 1–9 (2021). https://doi.org/10.3389/fpubh.2021.683712
79. Melin, J., Bonn, S. E., Pendrill, L., Trolle Lagerros, Y.: A questionnaire for assessing user satisfaction with mobile health apps: development using rasch measurement theory. JMIR Mhealth Uhealth, **8**(5), e15909(2020). https://doi.org/10.2196/15909
80. Azad-Khaneghah, P., Neubauer, N., Miguel Cruz, A., Liu, L.: Mobile health app usability and quality rating scales: a systematic review. Disabil. Rehabil.: Assist. Technol., **16**(7), 712–721(2021). https://doi.org/10.1080/17483107.2019.1701103
81. Fiore, P.: How to evaluate mobile health applications: A scoping review. In: Building capacity for health informatics in the future, vol. 234, (pp. 109–114), (2017). https://doi.org/10.3233/978-1-61499-742-9-109
82. Hermawati, S., Lawson, G.: Managing obesity through mobile phone applications: a state-of-the-art review from a user-centred design perspective. Pers. Ubiquit. Comput. **18**(8), 2003–2023 (2014). https://doi.org/10.1007/s00779-014-0757-4
83. Miralles, I., Granell, C.: Considerations for designing context-aware mobile apps for mental health interventions. Int. J. Environ. Res. Public Health **16**(7), 1197 (2019). https://doi.org/10.3390/ijerph16071197
84. Atchariyachanvanich, K., Mitinunwong, N., Tamthong, B.: Factors affecting disclosure of personal health information via mobile application. In: 2017 IEEE/ACIS 16th International conference on computer and information science (ICIS) (pp. 203–208), (2017). https://doi.org/10.1109/ICIS.2017.7959994
85. Lin, P.Y., Liang, T.P., Huang, H.C., Li, Y.W.: Design quality, relationship intimacy and continuance intention of mobile apps: an extension to the is success model. J. Electron. Commer. Res. **22**(4), 266–284 (2021)
86. Min, B.-W.: Improvement of mobile u-health services system. In: Communications in Computer and Information Science, vol. 262 CCIS, no. PART 1(pp. 44–51), (2011). https://doi.org/10.1007/978-3-642-27204-2_6

# Evaluation Review of Mobile Apps Supporting Adolescents' and Young Adults' Mental Health

**Milica Petrovic, Flavia Cristofolini, Marta Landoni, Chiara Ionio, and Andrea Gaggioli**

## 1 Introduction

Adolescence is a stage of life defined as a period between childhood and adulthood, with often no consensus regarding the age range [1]. The most common age range, also adopted by the authors of this chapter, for the adolescence (10–14) and young adult period (14–24) is between 10 and 24 [1]. The recognition of adolescence as a crucial period for the onset of mental health disorders has been growing in the past decade [2].

M. Petrovic · M. Landoni
Università Cattolica del Sacro Cuore, Milan, Italy
e-mail: milica.petrovic@unicatt.it

M. Petrovic
Department for Psychiatry, Psychosomatics and Psychotherapy, Goethe University, Depression Research Centre of the German Depression Foundation, Frankfurt, Germany

F. Cristofolini · A. Gaggioli (✉)
Research Center in Communication Psychology, Università Cattolica del Sacro Cuore, Milan, Italy
e-mail: andrea.gaggioli@unicatt.it

F. Cristofolini
e-mail: flavia.cristofolini@unicatt.it

C. Ionio
Centro Di Ricerca Sulle Dinamiche Evolutive Ed Educative, Università Cattolica del Sacro Cuore, CRIdeeMilan, Italy
e-mail: chiara.ionio@unicatt.it

F. Cristofolini · A. Gaggioli
IRCCS Istituto Auxologico Italiano, Milan, Italy

 
S. Scataglini et al. (eds.), *mHealth and Human-Centered Design Towards Enhanced Health, Care, and Well-Being*, Studies in Big Data 120,
https://doi.org/10.1007/978-981-99-3989-3_7

A systematic review [3] investigating secular trends in adolescents' mental health throughout the century concludes that internalizing symptoms have been continuously increasing. Such an increase is inevitably leading to difficulties in recognizing the adolescents and young adults in need of mental health support [2, 3].

Current estimates indicate that roughly 1 in 10 adolescents will experience a diagnosable mental health issue, while some studies pointed to a prevalence as high as 19% for mental health disorders among adolescents [4]. Additionally, COVID-19 has had a multifactorial impact on both children and adolescents [5]. For instance, it has been noted that stressors of the pandemic can potentially trigger neuroinflammation and behavioral impairments, while social isolation stress has a critical role in neuroimmunoendocrine changes during early age [5].

The wide use of technology among youth allows for new opportunities to reach out and integrate technology-based approaches into adolescents' health care [6]. Technology-based approaches, on the other hand, relate to methods for both diagnosis and therapy that communicate their messages via computers and mobile devices. [7]. Therefore, we distinguish the term *mHealth* in particular, which specifically addresses the use of mobile devices in delivering diagnostic and treatment strategies [8]. Mobile devices include mobile smartphones with wireless internet connection and access to mobile applications (i.e., apps). In line with that, the prevalence of smartphone ownership among adolescents is around 73%, while 92% of young adults report owning a cell phone [9]. In that sense, the current generation of adolescents and young adults can be distinguished as "always connected". Concretely, spending a significant amount of time online, using social media, YouTube, tweeting, or using other apps [6].

However, despite the rise in smartphone ownership among teenagers, there are few evidence-based mental health mobile apps currently on the market, and a lack of studies that bring together disorder-specific mental health apps for comparison. [10]. Moreover, the existing challenges of using mental health apps can be broadly categorized into (1) poor regulation of quality and privacy, (2) inconsistencies in engagement, and (3) narrow focus on one disorder per app [10–12].

Therefore, overcoming these challenges is more relevant than ever, and it requires a holistic approach to designing and developing new technology. Considering the environmental impact of humanity on a macro level, new developments require narrowing down and wisely distributing time and resources to each aspect of our existence. In such a way, the holistic approach would include the interventionists and/or designers, technologists, and stakeholders closely collaborating for the meaningful creation of technologies that will successfully serve the intended purpose.

Human-centered design (HCD) is an approach that bases product development on the information collected about the end-users and settings—i.e., the individuals the product is designed for [13]. HCD has a great potential in supporting complex health interventions simply by navigating population problems that often influence successful end-result [14]. In this manner, HCD can support the development of meaningful products and concretely purposeful and sustainable mobile apps for adolescents and young adults.

In this chapter, the existing mental health apps for adolescents and young adults are explored and assessed by utilizing the Evaluation Model Screener, which is a part of the American Psychiatric Association Comprehensive App Evaluation Model. Finally, reflections are made on the implications of HCD in mental health based on our example, and the chapter concludes with key considerations for the future developments of mHealth for adolescents and young adults.

## 2 Methods

Although the number of available apps for mental health is large, the evidence base is particularly scarce for adolescents [15]. Namely, a systematic review of mHealth apps for all ages has pointed out an important discrepancy between the development and research, with eight papers identified describing only five apps [16]. Furthermore, a review on mHealth by WHO identified 1536 apps for depression; however, only 32 of these were supported by published articles [17].

Interestingly, only few apps have been specifically developed for children and adolescents, but the concrete benefit of these apps remains unclear. For example, two systematic reviews [15, 18] exploring digital mental health interventions for children and young adults reveal that a randomized control trial (RCT) has been performed for only two apps. These RCTs showed no benefits of these apps on specific symptoms they were targeting.

Considering the scarce literature on evidence-based mHealth for adolescents and young adults, the authors performed a scoping review on the existing mental health apps for these populations. The American Psychiatric Assessment (APA) Framework Evaluation Model Screener (EMS) was used for the initial evaluation of the retrieved apps. The APA app evaluation model is applied to critically assess the quality of the app by taking into consideration accessibility, privacy and security, clinical foundation, engagement, and interoperability [19]. This model is addressing the urgent need for a comprehensible app evaluation tool that allows the assessment with a set of objective metrics. To this review, only the Evaluation Model Screener was used, which is the short version of the full framework and provides parameters for the initial assessment of an app with eight closed-ended questions (Table 2).

Our search strategy involved all relevant databases and additional search of other sources in line with our inclusion criteria. The apps included fit the age group of our interest (16–24) or can be applied to the age group of our interest. Some of the mobile applications included in the findings had set the age limit of 12+ although they focus on adolescents and young adults. Such apps were also considered relevant to the current search since a clear consensus about the age range for adolescence does not currently exist. Furthermore, the apps included had to be still available at the time the review was performed, active, and existing at least on one OS or platform. The apps that are not active anymore, or are not available in app stores or platforms, and are not available in English were excluded.

**Table 1** Search string and databases

| Databases | No. identified | No. retrieved | Final After Abstract/ Full text | Search string | Date |
|---|---|---|---|---|---|
| PubMed | 212 | 51 | 13 | ((mobile applications) AND (mental health)) AND (young people/young adults) | 2000–2022 |
| Psych INFO | 2 | 1 | 0 | Mobile apps AND mental health AND youth | 2000–2022 |
| CENTRAL | 26 | 6 | 1 | Mobile apps AND mental health AND youth | 2000–2022 |
| Scopus | 174 | 21 | 4 | Mobile apps AND mental health AND youth | 2000–2022 |

The assessment included all relevant literature that (1) evaluated mental health apps for (2) young people from the age of sixteen until the age of 24, or can be applied to young people, that address (3) mental health issues and promote psychological well-being (4) published in English/available in English (5) from the year of 2000 up to date.

Excluded literature addressed mental health apps for youth (1) with no concrete model, approach, or framework and (2) did not provide evidence or rationale for the creation/use of the concrete app. Furthermore, papers that are (3) not published in English were excluded. Our keywords included: Mobile apps, mental health apps, youth, adolescents, and young adults. The search was completed in January 2022 (Table 1).

## 3 Evaluation Results

Eighteen mental health apps for supporting adolescent and young adults were retrieved. The apps included were ClinTouch (ClinTouchSWL), JoyPop, iBobbly, Psychologist in a pocket (PiaP), BlueIce, MindClimb, MindSurf, Music eScape, PRIME, SleepNinja, MyMoodCoach, Niggle, Calm, WeClick, Stop Breathe Think, Headspace, Nod, and CatchIt.

Table 3 summarizes the results of the evaluation of the selected applications, based on the mental health domain chosen and of the underlying approaches and principles, while the first evaluation of these apps against the APA EMS questions is presented in Table 4.

The APA EMS questions offer an initial evaluation of the mHealth apps based on the OS, the regularity of the updates, transparency with the privacy policy, sensitive data management, research and evidence basis, clinical/recovery foundation, usability, and the alignment of the app with the stated purpose. Upon the initial evaluation, which is the simplified version of the full evaluation, the apps with higher

**Table 2** List of apps and Evaluation model screener score

| Apps | APA EMS (Yes/No) | APA EMS Sample |
|---|---|---|
| ClinTouch | 7/1 | 1. On which platform/operating system does the app work?<br>2. Has the app been updated in the last 180 days?<br>3. Is there a transparent privacy policy that is clear and accessible before use?<br>4. Does the app, collect, use, and/or transmit sensitive data? If yes, does it claim to do so securely?<br>5. Is there evidence of specific benefit from academic institutions, end-user feedback, or research studies?<br>6. Does the app have clinical/recovery foundation relevant to your intended use?<br>7. Does the app seem easy to use?<br>8. Can data be easily shared and interpreted in a way that's consistent with the stated purpose of the app? |
| PRIME | 4/4 | |
| JoyPop | 6/2 | |
| Niggle | 6/2 | |
| WeClick | 4/4 | |
| Music eScape | 6/2 | |
| iBobbly | 7/1 | |
| BlueIce | 6/2 | |
| PiaP | 4/4 | |
| Nod | 7/1 | |
| MindClimb | 6/2 | |
| MindSurf | 6/2 | |
| MyMoodCoach | 6/2 | |
| CatchIt | 5/3 | |
| SleepNinja | 8/0 | |
| Calm | 8/0 | |
| Stop Breathe Think | 7/1 | |
| HeadSpace | 8/0 | |

scores can also be evaluated against the full APA Comprehensive Evaluation Model. However, a clear guideline is not provided regarding the APA EMS scores, therefore we argue that 4/4 should be considered a lower limit for further consideration of an app for detailed evaluation, while the 8/0 score should be interpreted as an excellent screener score, encouraging detailed app evaluation using the full Comprehensive Evaluation Model. Following the obtained score in our evaluation, we can argue that the retrieved apps vary in the initial assessment quality from high quality to medium quality, with one app reaching the lower limit for further consideration.

Most retrieved apps focus on limited and specific mental health issues of adolescents and young adults such as stress, anxiety, depression, psychosis, suicidal ideation, schizophrenia, etc. They offer a range of support mechanisms such as symptom tracking, self-assessment, journaling, mood mapping, social networking and connection with peers, well-being podcasts and quizzes, meditation, and peer feedback. A full list of clinical goals that these mental health apps for adolescents address includes: tracking and assisting with the management of psychotic symptoms (ClinTouch) and improving the quality of life of people living with schizophrenia (PRIME), offering skills for suicide prevention and reduction of self-harm behaviors (iBobbly, BlueIce), depression treatment (PiaP, Nod), coping with psychological distress, anxiety, and poor mental health (MindClimb, MindSurf, MyMoodCoach,

**Table 3** Summary of the retrieved apps

| App | Mental health domains | Support function | Approaches and principles |
|---|---|---|---|
| Clin Touch | Psychosis | Assists users to keep track of their psychotic symptoms. The app asks users to rate their experience a few times per day and provides real-time illness management solutions | CBT approach |
| iBobbly | Suicide prevention | The app walks the user through the self-assessment and then provides feedback, with an option of keeping a mood diary. It helps users learn how to manage feelings and thoughts (including suicidal thoughts) with an automatic routing to emergency phone numbers | Emotion awareness and regulation |
| PiaP | Depression | The PiaP app analyzes how the user writes (following DSM-IV guidelines), says things, and how often he/she leaves the house. Additionally, it allows the EEG consumer devices to analyze the users' psychological responses, particularly the exposition therapy and journaling session | CBT approach, peer feedback, narrative principles in therapy |
| BlueIce | Self-harm behaviors | A prescribed evidence-based app aiming to reduce self-harm behaviors in young people and support emotion management. The app consists of a mood diary, a toolkit to reduce distress, and automatic routing to emergency numbers, if urges to harm, do not cease | Emotion awareness and regulation |

(continued)

**Table 3** (continued)

| App | Mental health domains | Support function | Approaches and principles |
|---|---|---|---|
| The MindClimb | Anxiety | The app is designed to assist users with anxiety throughout cognitive behavioral therapy, and it can be used simultaneously during therapy | CBT approach, interactive storytelling |
| MindSurf | Stress | The app trains self-help strategies, promotes contentment, well-being, and goal achievement by assisting with the resolution of internal conflicts underlying psychological distress | Method of Levels (MOL) Transdiagnostic Cognitive Therapy |
| PRIME | Schizophrenia | The app aims to improve the quality of life of people living with schizophrenia. It enables social networking with peers who experience similar difficulties, supports setting goals, and enables getting in touch with mental health coaches in the area | CBT approach, peer support |
| SleepNinja | Sleep quality | This app draws from CBT-I to teach users strategies to improve their sleep | CBT approach |
| Niggle | Psychological distress | It helps youth understand, capture, and keep track of their "niggles, that is moderate symptoms of discomfort and anxiety". In essence, the app acts as a preventive tool that assists young people to understand how to manage adverse emotions, through watching supporting videos, listening to podcasts, and partaking in quizzes | Emotion awareness and regulation |

(continued)

CatchIt, WeClick), sleep improvement (Sleep Ninja). A smaller group of apps focus on enhancing adolescents' well-being and their positive psychological functioning, mainly through improving and supporting emotional awareness (JoyPop, Niggle, WeClick, Music eScape), and supporting mindfulness practice (Calm, Stop Breathe Think, HeadSpace).

**Table 3** (continued)

| App | Mental health domains | Support function | Approaches and principles |
|---|---|---|---|
| Nod | Loneliness and depression | This app is designed to help college students manage loneliness and depression by building social connections through small and achievable steps, in-app exercises, and peer perspectives and feedback | CBT approach, peer support, narrative principles in therapy |
| WeClick | Improving relationships issues | The app is based on the CBT principles and the Social Learning model. WeClick app is an interactive storytelling app following four characters that share stories about different problems | CBT approach; Social Learning model; peer support; narrative principles in therapy |
| CatchIt | Adverse emotions | This app is designed following CBT principles, aiming to assist users to manage feelings of anxiety, depression, confusion, and anger by training self-help strategies | CBT approach, interactive storytelling |
| **WELL-BEING APPS** | | | |
| Music eScape | Emotional competence | The app analyzes songs in users' libraries in line with their level of valence (pleasant to unpleasant) and arousal (very low to very high) by using The Echo Nest music data program. The songs are then sorted in two-dimensional space and divided according to Russel's circumplex model of emotion and labeled. The user then has access to the mood map of their music (i.e., the eScape) | Emotion awareness and regulation; Russel's circumplex model of emotion; The Echo Nest music data program |

(continued)

The prevailing theoretical framework of apps focusing on clinical disorders and symptoms is CBT, while other psychological theories, such as attachment theories or ACT, are lacking; a wider range of approaches should be explored to offer increasingly effective tools for therapeutic change via mobile apps.

**Table 3** (continued)

| App | Mental health domains | Support function | Approaches and principles |
|---|---|---|---|
| JoyPop | Emotional competence; Optimism training | Users are asked to complete MoodRating each day, and if happiness rates are less than 50%, then they are asked to rate how sad, angry, or "meh" they are feeling. In this manner, they have an opportunity to identify negative emotions, which promotes emotional awareness. If mood ratings are negative, the users are redirected to an activity to help them shift their mindset toward positive emotions | Emotion awareness and regulation; Positive Psychology; |
| MyMoodCoach | Well-being and poor mental health prevention | The app targets the prevention of poor mental health and promotion of well-being in young adults by training self-help strategies that can reduce worry or boredom and increase self-confidence, optimism, motivation, and recognition and understanding of emotions | CBT approach, Positive Psychology, interactive storytelling |
| Calm | Well-being- Meditation and Mindfulness | The app promotes well-being through meditation and mindfulness. The included app topics cover anxiety, stress, sleep disturbances, self-esteem, happiness, focus, etc | Mindfulness-based Stress Reduction Mindfulness-based Cognitive Therapy |
| Stop breathe think | Well-being-mindfulness | This is a mindfulness-based app that supports meditation techniques and assists users to maintain their mindfulness practice | Mindfulness-based Stress Reduction Mindfulness-based Cognitive Therapy |
| Headspace | Well-being-Meditation practices | This is a mindfulness meditation-based app that provides guided and unguided meditation | Mindfulness-based Stress Reduction Mindfulness-based Cognitive Therapy |

**Table 4** Positive technology apps

| Apps | Determinants of personal experience | Key factors | Strategies |
|---|---|---|---|
| JoyPop | Eudaimonic level | Resilience, emotion regulation skills, self-empathy (emotional awareness) | Journal feature to record thoughts and feelings; prompts to distract from negative to positive emotionality; breathing exercises |
| Stop Breathe Think | Hedonic level | Mindfulness | MBSR strategies |
| Headspace | Hedonic level | Mindfulness, Meditation | Guided mindfulness meditations, mindful breathing, sitting meditation, body check (focusing on certain body parts), spatial focus (fixed vs. moving), and aperture of attention (narrow vs. diffuse) |
| Calm | Hedonic level | Meditation, mindfulness, | Audio-guided contents: soundscapes, sleeping stories, music |
| MyMoodCoach | Eudaimonic level | Self-Efficacy and motivation | Emotion Diary; motivation, confidence, optimism strategies |

The prevalence of issue-focused mental health apps over the well-being-focused apps echoes a consideration of mental health only in relation to psychological difficulties or diagnosis of a mental illness. However, according to WHO [20], mental health should be regarded as the capacity to be productive and make a positive contribution to society rather than the absence of particular issues. Specifically, WHO introduced the concept of Positive Mental Health, defined as "*a positive emotion (affect) such as feelings of happiness, a personality trait inclusive of the psychological resources of self-esteem and mastery, and as resilience, which is the capacity to cope with adversity*" [21]. Therefore, the concept of well-being goes beyond the absence of mental health disorders and symptoms: it encompasses subjective well-being, positive relationships, and personal growth [22, 23].

Our analysis seems to indicate that Positive Psychology, which has been offering a deeper understanding of psychological well-being for at least two decades, is only partially inspiring mHealth tools: 2 apps out of 18 contain Positive Psychology factors such as optimism (myMoodCoach) and positive emotions (JoyPop), although in both cases only as part of a wider range of goals including also psychological distress. No app among these supports the user to only enhance his/her positive mental health and well-being. The rest of the well-being apps within our analysis promote mostly emotion awareness and regulation through Mood tracking, Mood reflection, Mindfulness, and Meditation.

Interestingly, there is an evident lack of consensus over the full definition of digital health that specifically aims at well-being and self-empowerment. Some authors [24] define well-being apps as "promotion and prevention apps", meant to promote strengths and thus also prevent mental illness. The authors choose here to refer "well-being apps" in relation to the framework of Positive Technology [25], which studies technologies aimed specifically at supporting well-being and fostering the growth of individuals, groups, and institutions. Positive Technologies encompass a wide range of domains, including mental health, but also neurorehabilitation/cognitive enhancement, multicultural integration, socio-cognitive skills, and education. Considering that well-being is per se subjective and therefore too vague for a scientific context, the authors chose to adopt here the analysis focus of "personal experience" present in the Positive Technology framework [26].

More precisely, the evaluation of the apps for well-being is based on how they induce positive and pleasant experiences (i.e., emotional quality, the *Hedonic* component), support individuals in reaching engaging and self-actualizing experiences (i.e., the *Eudaimonic* component) and promote social/Interpersonal relationships (*Connectedness*). Based on this framework, among the apps that have been analyzed, the following (Table 4) may be considered as Positive Technologies; for each, the evaluation is suggested based on the model:

The apps focusing on emotional awareness can be considered as Positive Technologies because they facilitate emotion regulation, which can be considered an underlying factor to achieve positive mental health and well-being [27]. Most hedonic apps in this analysis support the hypothesis that how technology is built to enhance well-being can go beyond simply the momentary hedonic experience to include its longer-term eudaimonia. [25].

In the effort of applying an overall framework to the evaluation of mHealth youth apps, inclusive of the recent definition of mental health, a distinction was made between (1) mental health apps aimed at decreasing psychological distress and specific clinical disorders, (2) well-being apps aimed at promoting positive mental health and emotional awareness (thus belonging to the Positive Technologies).

However, considering the multidimensional nature of well-being [28], it is becoming important to understand what well-being means to adolescents [29], as this has evident implications for the development not only of tools to measure their well-being and but also of mHealth apps. Adolescents' perceptions of their own well-being differ from adults [30], therefore adult—only based research must be integrated with adolescents' views [31, 32]. Some authors compared the conceptualization of well-being of expert practitioners and researchers with the one of British young people aged 11–16. Findings revealed crucial differences: for example, young people highly valued the role of external influences on their well-being, parents', and friends', both positively, as fulfillment of acceptance and belonging needs, and negatively, as resistance to others' judgment. This is explained by young people's life experience of still being reliant on others while adults are more independent.

As regards happiness and flourishing, young people identified "feeling good" not only with positive feelings but also with having a purpose in life and achieving of their purpose. A first tentative definition of well-being from these adolescents' point of view is summarized by the authors as "multifaceted perception of an interaction between an individual's positive feelings and external influences".

These and further related findings will have to inform youth participatory approaches and youth-centered design of mHealth well-being and mental health tools.

## 4 The Role Of Human-Centered Design in mHealth Apps

The traditional technology-driven approach to the development of computer systems has been a primary method of creating technological advances. In this approach, the human factor was a matter of adaptation rather than the focus [33]. It can be suggested that mastering technological development came at the price of neglecting the actual user. However, contemporary implementation practice has prioritized users as the focal point of technological progress [13]. Human-centered design allows a more enduring approach to modeling users' behavior, resulting in intuitive interfaces, easier understanding, and fewer performance errors [33].

HCD is deeply rooted in psychological theory (e.g., cognitive psychology, organizational psychology, social psychology) and can be a potential solution to the common struggle of psychologists to implement generated mental health knowledge in a meaningful and sustainable manner [33, 34]. More specifically, HCD is not a method, but rather a field that is utilizing different research methodologies to align the products with the context of their intended use [35].

Human-centered design is commonly used in the development of digital technologies [35], but interestingly, it has also been used for non-technological problems such as improving school lunches [35, 36], improving the patient-healthcare experience [37], and advancing mental health services [38]. In fact, "Software psychology" was first used in 1970 to describe the shift to consideration of human characteristics and needs as a focal point of technological development [39].

In health practice, HCD includes the three-part cyclical process that enables the stakeholders to understand the needs and challenges of end-users, produce ideas and solutions based on those needs, and complete the implementation of health strategies [14]. Interestingly, especially in digital mental health development, content development occurs separately from technology development [40], which inevitably influences and hinders user experience. More specifically, numerous existing models that guide the design of digital health interventions are based on an outdated understanding of the data available and limited interaction points with end-users [40]. Moreover, in digital health collaborations, it is a common practice for mental health experts to develop content while the developers design the app independently. On the other hand, mobile apps on some occasions deliver rather static interventions without any personalization available or further considerations of how the specific app can be adapted for the end-users.

The gap in user involvement for product development can also be demonstrated by drawing a parallel between the retrieved apps and the literature that reflects on the reported adolescent's needs and feedback gathered regarding the mHealth and eHealth development. Although the apps we distinguished from the literature are validated and address relevant mental health issues of adolescents, the user interface aspects might still not correspond to the end-user needs, which will ultimately influence app usage. For instance, in a study exploring the design features of effective eHealth [41], it was noted that social context and support, contact with intervention, tailoring or personalization option as well as the support of self-management are important aspects distinguished by the end-users.

Moreover, adolescents highlight that the intervention needs to respect their individuality [42], and communicate important concepts avoiding instructive nature (e.g., "*We think that adults are just gonna change our decisions—and we're really scared of that 'cause we wanna stay the way we are*" pp. 3334 [42]). Interestingly, the adolescents also note they would benefit from confidence-boosting and supportive content, as well as inspiration, and discussions on the pros/cons of specific behavioral responses [43]. The content that was informative rather than patronizing is perceived as more beneficial, while the support of peers was considered more important than the support of mental health practitioners [44].

We must note that while prioritizing user needs should be the focus in HCD, too much complexity or integration of numerous ideas within one app can be a similar drawback as the previously mentioned issue of static interventions. In fact, a great minimum viable product is often better, user experience wise, than an overly complex one [45].

Moreover, besides HCD, it must also be noted that the rapid technological evolution towards more intelligent interactive technologies poses seven grand challenges in terms of human–computer interaction (HCI), and technology's impact on individuals and societies [46]. These challenges are beyond the design and development focus and include Human-Technology Symbiosis, Human–Environment Interactions, Ethics, Privacy and Security, Well-being, Health and Eudaimonia, Accessibility and Universal Access, Learning and Creativity, and Social Organization and Democracy [46].

In fact, these HCI challenges must be considered and reflected in HCD so that rather than designing technological solutions that will encounter these challenges, we work on the creation of technology that is able to overcome such challenges as they arise. So far, these important HCD considerations are notably lacking in the existing mental health apps for adolescents and arguably HCD is widely neglected. While the existing apps are mainly disorder-treatment focused, the user-centered considerations that align user needs throughout the disorders are missing. Ultimately this leads to user experience issues and app dropout, resulting in the aggregation of design, development, and technology of no use.

## 5 Conclusions

This review provided an insight into the existing validated mental health apps for adolescents and young adults that can support mental health and provide both some support for the psychological issues and enhancement of well-being.

It must be noted that limiting the search to available apps in English has narrowed down the findings, and likely excluded other valuable apps available. However, interpretations and significant conclusions can still be made based on the retrieved apps. Namely, although the existing apps address a range of issues, it must be noted that (1) some of these apps are not simultaneously available on both Android and iPhone IOS; (2) the narrow focus on specific mental issues requires users to understand personal mental health and problems they are experiencing in order to search for the concrete app, which might be difficult for children and adolescents but also creates the need to access multiple apps for different issues; and finally, (3) these apps are available among numerous other apps that claim to address similar issues with no research to support such claims. Therefore, it might be difficult for the user to distinguish apps that are going to be helpful.

Following these conclusions, we argue that the optimal mental health app for adolescents and young adults should be readily available on both operating systems, allowing easy access. Moreover, the optimal app inevitably must support general well-being with built-in screening that will allow necessary personalization to direct users to required support with no prior knowledge of mental health (e.g., different support mechanisms for different issues). In this manner, the app facilitates recognition of potential issues and navigates the user to proper tools that can support and help him/her manage these issues, rather than requiring the user to know the issues beforehand or in some instances even have an advanced understanding of the issue before any contact with the app. Additionally, the optimal mental health app needs to be created following a human-centered design approach, allowing the user's involvement in the app creation, while offering skill training for decreasing mental health issues but also enhancing positive mental health and well-being. Finally, well-being features should offer eudaimonic and connection-based experiences and not only hedonic/emotional experiences. Human-centered design allows a more enduring approach to modeling users' behavior, resulting in intuitive interfaces, easier understanding, and fewer performance errors [33].

**Acknowledgements** This research was partially supported by the KA220-YOU—Cooperation partnerships in youth "E+Wellbeing App".

## References

1. Sawyer, S.M., Azzopardi, P.S., Wickremarathne, D., Patton, G.C.: The age of adolescence. Lancet Child & Adolesc. Health. **2**(3), 223–228 (2018)

2. Patalay, P., Gage, S.H.: Changes in millennial adolescent mental health and health-related behaviours over 10 years: a population cohort comparison study. Int. J. Epidemiol. **48**(5), 1650–1664 (2019)
3. Bor, W., Dean, A.J., Najman, J., Hayatbakhsh, R.: Are child and adolescent mental health problems increasing in the 21st century? A systematic review. Aust. N. Z. J. Psychiatry **48**(7), 606–616 (2014)
4. Fink, E., Patalay, P., Sharpe, H., Holley, S., Deighton, J., Wolpert, M.: Mental health difficulties in early adolescence: a comparison of two cross-sectional studies in England from 2009 to 2014. J. Adolesc. Health **56**(5), 502–507 (2015)
5. de Figueiredo, C.S., Sandre, P.C., Portugal, L.C., Mázala-de-Oliveira, T., da Silva, C.L., Raony, Í., Ferreira, E.S., Giestal-de-Araujo, E., Dos Santos, A.A., Bomfim, P.O.: COVID-19 pandemic impact on children and adolescents' mental health: Biological, environmental, and social factors. Prog. Neuropsychopharmacol. Biol. Psychiatry **2**(106), 110171 (2021)
6. Radovic, A., McCarty, C.A., Katzman, K., Richardson, L.P.: Adolescents' perspectives on using technology for health: qualitative study. JMIR Pediatr. Parent. **1**(1), e8677 (2018)
7. Carreiro, S., Chai, P.R., Carey, J., Lai, J., Smelson, D., Boyer, E.W.: mHealth for the detection and intervention in adolescent and young adult substance use disorder. Curr. Addict. Rep. **5**(2), 110–119 (2018)
8. Gaggioli, A., Riva, G.: From mobile mental health to mobile wellbeing: opportunities and challenges. Stud. Health Technol. Inform **184**, 141–147 (2013)
9. Lenhart, A.: Teens, social media & technology overview 2015. (2015). Accessed from https://www.pewresearch.org/internet/2015/04/09/teens-social-media-technology-2015/ (April, 2022).
10. Chandrashekar, P.: Do mental health mobile apps work: evidence and recommendations for designing high-efficacy mental health mobile apps. Mhealth., **4**, (2018)
11. Marley, J., Farooq, S.: Mobile telephone apps in mental health practice: uses, opportunities and challenges. BJPsych bulletin. **39**(6), 288–290 (2015)
12. Leigh, S., Flatt, S.: App-based psychological interventions: friend or foe? Evid. Based Ment. Health **18**(4), 97–99 (2015)
13. Lyon, A.R., Brewer, S.K., Areán, P.A.: Leveraging human-centered design to implement modern psychological science: Return on an early investment. Am. Psychol. **75**(8), 1067 (2020)
14. Adam, M.B., Minyenya-Njuguna, J., Karuri Kamiru, W., Mbugua, S., Makobu, N.W., Donelson, A.J.: Implementation research and human-centred design: how theory driven human-centred design can sustain trust in complex health systems, support measurement and drive sustained community health volunteer engagement. Health Policy Plan., **35**(Supplement_2), ii150-ii162 (2020).
15. Grist, R., Porter, J., Stallard, P.: Mental health mobile apps for preadolescents and adolescents: a systematic review. J. Med. Internet Res. **19**(5), e7332 (2017)
16. Donker, T., Petrie, K., Proudfoot, J., Clarke, J., Birch, M.R., Christensen, H.: Smartphones for smarter delivery of mental health programs: a systematic review. J. Med. Internet Res. **15**(11), e2791 (2013)
17. Martínez-Pérez, B., De La Torre-Díez, I., López-Coronado, M.: Mobile health applications for the most prevalent conditions by the World Health Organization: review and analysis. J. Med. Internet Res. **15**(6), e2600 (2013)
18. Hollis, C., Falconer, C.J., Martin, J.L., Whittington, C., Stockton, S., Glazebrook, C., Davies, E.B.: Annual research review: digital health interventions for children and young people with mental health problems–a systematic and meta-review. J. Child Psychol. Psychiatry **58**(4), 474–503 (2017)
19. Lagan, S., Aquino, P., Emerson, M.R., Fortuna, K., Walker, R., Torous, J.: Actionable health app evaluation: translating expert frameworks into objective metrics. NPJ digital medicine. **3**(1), 1–8 (2020)
20. World Health Organization. Promoting mental health: concepts, emerging evidence, practice (Summary Report). World Health Organization, Geneva (2004)

21. World Health Organization.: Promoting mental health: concepts, emerging evidence, practice: a report of the World Health Organization, Department of Mental Health and Substance Abuse in collaboration with the Victorian Health Promotion Foundation and the University of Melbourne. World Health Organization, (2005). https://apps.who.int/iris/handle/10665/43286
22. Deci, E.L., Ryan, R.M.: Hedonia, eudaimonia, and well-being: An introduction. J. Happiness Stud. **9**(1), 1–1 (2008)
23. Keyes, C.L.: The mental health continuum: From languishing to flourishing in life. J. Health Soc. Behav. **1**, 207–222 (2002)
24. Michel, T., Tachtler, F., Slovak, P., Fitzpatrick, G.A.: Review of youth mental health promotion apps towards their fit with youth media preferences. EAI Endorsed Trans. Pervasive Health Technol., **5**(17), (2019)
25. Gaggioli, A., Riva, G., Peters, D., Calvo, R.A.: Positive Technology, computing, and design: shaping a future in which technology promotes psychological well-being. In: Emotions and Affect in Human Factors and Human–Computer Interaction (pp. 477–502). (2017)
26. Villani, D., Cipresso, P., Gaggioli, A., Riva, G.: Integrating technology in positive psychology practice. IGI Global, Hershey, PA (2016). https://doi.org/10.4018/978-1-4666-9986-1
27. Peters, D., Calvo, R.A., Ryan, R.M.: Designing for motivation, engagement and wellbeing in digital experience. Front. Psychol. **28**(9), 797 (2018)
28. Ross, D.A., Hinton, R., Melles-Brewer, M., Engel, D., Zeck, W., Fagan, L., Herat, J., Phaladi, G., Imbago-Jácome, D., Anyona, P., Sanchez, A., Damji, N., Terki, F., Baltag, V., Patton, G., Silverman, A., Fogstad, H., Banerjee, A., Mohan, A.: Adolescent well-being: a definition and conceptual framework. J. Adolesc. Health: Off. Publ. Soc. Adolesc. Med. **67**(4), 472–476 (2020). https://doi.org/10.1016/j.jadohealth.2020.06.042
29. Alexandrova, A.: A Philosophy for the Science of Wellbeing. Oxford University Press, United States of America (2017). https://doi.org/10.1093/oso/9780199300518.001.0001
30. Gillett-Swan, J.K.: Investigating tween children's capacity to conceptualise the complex issue of wellbeing. Glob. Stud. Child. **4**(2), 64–76 (2014)
31. Gennings, E., Brown, H.J., Hewlett, D.: (Constructing a definition: adolescent wellbeing from the perspective of the child and expert. Int. J. Wellbeing **11**(1), 69–88 (2021). https://doi.org/10.5502/ijw.v11i1.146)
32. Bharara, G., Duncan, S., Jarden, A., Hinckson, E.: A prototype analysis of New Zealand adolescents' conceptualizations of wellbeing. Int J Wellbeing **9**(4), 1–25 (2019). https://doi.org/10.5502/ijw.v9i4.975
33. Oviatt, S.: Human-centered design meets cognitive load theory: designing interfaces that help people think. In: Proceedings of the 14th ACM international conference on Multimedia (pp. 871–880), (2006)
34. Chambers, D.A.: Advancing the science of implementation: A workshop summary. Adm. Policy Ment. Health Ment. Health Serv. Research. **35**(1), 3–10 (2008)
35. Albert, B., Tullis, T.: Measuring the user experience: collecting, analyzing, and presenting usability metrics, pp. 100−113. Newnes, (2013)
36. Kalil, T.: Using human-centered design to make government work better and cost less. The White House, (2015)
37. Harte, R., Glynn, L., Rodríguez-Molinero, A., Baker, P.M., Scharf, T., Quinlan, L.R., Ólaighin, G.: A human-centered design methodology to enhance the usability, human factors, and user experience of connected health systems: a three-phase methodology. JMIR Hum. Factors **4**(1), e5443 (2017)
38. Lyon, A.R., Munson, S.A., Renn, B.N., Atkins, D.C., Pullmann, M.D., Friedman, E., Areán, P.A.: Use of human-centered design to improve implementation of evidence-based psychotherapies in low-resource communities: protocol for studies applying a framework to assess usability. JMIR Res. Protoc. **8**(10), e14990 (2019)
39. Shneiderman, B.: Software psychology: Human factors in com. Winthrop Publishers, Computer and Information Systems, Cambridge, Massachusetts, USA (1980)
40. Lyon, A.R., Dopp, A.R., Brewer, S.K., Kientz, J.A., Munson, S.A.: Designing the future of children's mental health services. Administration and Policy in Mental Health and Mental Health Services Research. **47**(5), 735–751 (2020)

41. Morrison, L.G., Yardley, L., Powell, J., Michie, S.: What design features are used in effective e-health interventions? A review using techniques from critical interpretive synthesis. Telemed. E-Health. **18**(2), 137–144 (2012)
42. Ranney, M.L., Pittman, S.K., Riese, A., Ybarra, M., Huang, J., Spirito, A., Rosen, R.: Mobile health intervention development principles: lessons from an adolescent cyberbullying intervention. In: Proceedings of the 51st Hawaii International conference on system sciences (2018)
43. O'Brien, K.H., Wyman Battalen, A., Sellers, C.M., Spirito, A., Yen, S., Maneta, E., Ryan, C.A., Braciszewski, J.M.: An mHealth approach to extend a brief intervention for adolescent alcohol use and suicidal behavior: Qualitative analyses of adolescent and parent feedback. J. Technol. Hum. Serv. **37**(4), 255–285 (2019)
44. mHealth Can Help Teens, Young adults struggling with depression. Accessed from https://mhealthintelligence.com/news/mhealth-can-help-teens-young-adults-struggling-with-depression
45. Schuh, G., Dölle, C., Schloesser, S.: Agile Prototyping for technical systems–Towards an adaption of the minimum viable product principle. DS 91: Proceedings of NordDesign 2018. Linköping, Sweden (2018)
46. Stephanidis, C., Salvendy, G., Antona, M., Chen, J.Y., Dong, J., Duffy, V.G., Fang, X., Fidopiastis, C., Fragomeni, G., Fu, L.P., Guo, Y.: Seven HCI grand challenges. Int. J. Hum.-Comput. Interaction. **35**(14), 1229–1269 (2019)

# An Overview of the Effects of Music on Tourette Syndrome

**Scataglini Sofia**

## 1 Introduction

Tourette Syndrome (TS) is a neurodevelopmental disorder with motor and vocal tics [1]. Head jerking, eye blinking, shoulder shrugs, and other body movements are examples of motor tics, while vocal tics include barks, grunts, yelps, and coughs [2]. Because TS is a comorbid disorder, symptoms may also include obsessive–compulsive disorder or attention deficit hyperactivity disorder (ADHD) [2]. There are several treatments for TS, the most common of which is pharmacotherapy [3], which has strong, modest, and empirical support. However, current treatments for TS either have side effects for patients or do not have long-term effects [4]. Tics have been studied because they can be caused by stressors as well as positive and negative emotions [5]. Several types of therapies have been used to test the efficacy of TS over time. Clinical assessment of TS-related symptoms necessitates a multidisciplinary approach that allows for a qualitative or partially quantitative evaluation of the subject using standard clinical scales following a clinical examination or video recording. Recent technological advancements have resulted in the development of new clinical practice systems capable of measuring important human movement parameters, such as quantifying bradykinesia and dyskinesia in neurological illnesses such as Parkinson's Disease using wearable devices. Music has been shown to have a therapeutic effect on neurological disorders [6]. Tics frequency appears to be influenced by a combination of motor imagery and musical imagery [5]. Motor imagery has been shown to help patients with movement disorders improve their motor performance. There is a correlation between the brain regions that are active when performing an action and those that are active when visualizing that action. Page et al. [7] compared

S. Sofia (✉)
Faculty of Medicine and Health Sciences, Dept. of Rehabilitation Sciences and Physiotherapy, Antwerp, Belgium
e-mail: sofia.scataglini@uantwerpen.be



S. Scataglini et al. (eds.), *mHealth and Human-Centered Design Towards Enhanced Health, Care, and Well-Being*, Studies in Big Data 120,
https://doi.org/10.1007/978-981-99-3989-3_8

the effectiveness of an occupational therapy-only rehabilitation program with one that also included creative assignments [7]. For six weeks, patients employed motor imagery for ten minutes twice a week at home and three times a week following each therapy session. Each patient's motor performance was enhanced by the motor imagery [7]. It has been demonstrated that music affects TS patients, specifically their tics [8]. In a case study utilizing wearable technology, Scataglini et al. [9] investigated the impact of rhythmic auditory stimulation (RAS) on the modulation of tics in TS. The procedure involved simultaneously recording footage from a camera and synchronized tic detection recordings from a wearable device placed on the patient's trunk. Data integration as a video and acceleration signal for assessing intensity and frequency using a five-level scale was done using the Advene Software package [11]. Music was played both at home and in hospital settings, both with and without earphones and in and out of the examiner's presence. The findings showed that 4/4 rhythmic auditory stimulation lessened the frequency of high-intensity tics. In particular, listening to the same music using earphones results in a 67% reduction [9, 10]. Due to the COVID-19 epidemic, a concern has recently been raised about whether it is possible to monitor the impact of music on TS without a wearable device and in close proximity to the patient. This chapter will provide an overview of how music affects TS while examining the connections between music, musicians, and TS that provide mHealth and telehealth services.

## *1.1 Effect of Music in Neurology and Particular in TS*

Music therapy is used to treat various diseases, including TS and Parkinson's Disease (PD). Thaut et al. (2019) conducted a study on Parkinson's disease patients, many of whom exhibit bradykinesia, tremor, and impaired posture and balance. Listening to music with rhythmic signals can help the brain anticipate movement, which aids in movement coordination. The experimental group in the study received rhythmic auditory stimulation (RAS) training for 30 min each day. The study found that RAS improves gait parameters in Parkinson's disease patients [12]. Pohl et al. (2013) tested the effect of active music therapy on cognition with a neurological examination [13]. The results showed an improvement in verbal memory, language, function, and attention. Other mental studies with music therapy focused on the mood of patients. Studies showed a decrease in depression, emotions, self-esteem, and social isolation, while other studies showed no improvement [13]. Music has been demonstrated to improve brain neuronal connections [14]. A study was conducted that largely focused on tics and music, evaluating the influence of music on tics and the factors that lead to tic reduction [8]. The subjects were initially given a questionnaire to fill out on how their tics changed while listening to music, performing, and singing. Patients were videotaped in a room as they played or sang their chosen piece of music, listened to music, and used mental imagery of musical performance, and their results were compared to a baseline [8]. People with TS tend to be more creative than healthy people [15]. This skill and motor energy can be applied to functional activities that can aid in the reduction of tics. These skill activities may include musical activities, which are advantageous since music allows for more rhythmic motions [5]. Music can improve coordination and precision, which can help to minimize the involuntary movements induced by tics [5]. Music can be utilized as a treatment tool to activate a psychophysiological state, an emotion, or to use in interventions [16]. It can also help express feelings and thoughts that were previously suppressed verbally. Listening to music on a daily basis has been shown to help stroke patients recover [5]. Music can also have a significant impact on mood. Pleasure studies with specific musical songs can influence a person's mood and feelings, as well as the intensity of tics when involving TS [5]. In light of this, a study was designed to discover how music and motor activities affect patients' tics and mood [5]. A pilot study was conducted using an intervention called "Imagine, Tourette!" that included dancing with and without music as well as motor imagery exercises [5]. There were eight patients (six males and two females) from the Italian region between the ages of 20 and 35 with TS. Patients had cognitive-behavioral psychotherapy for 4 months. Two well-known songs were selected: "Gioca Jouer" by Cecchetto [17] and "Testa-spalla" by Don Lurio [18]. Two songs were chosen to reduce the possibility of negative emotions due to personal preference. A psychologist administered exams to participants before, during, and after the creation. The intervention consisted of eight 15-min sessions delivered online using cameras over the course of two weeks. Trainers and patients were both alone in quiet offices or homes. The trainers were two TS experts. The experimental group performed motor activities while listening to music, while the control group completed the identical activities without listening to music. The experimental group viewed a music video containing choreography and then performed the actions while watching the video again. The control group did the same thing as the experimental group, but without music. Every one of the eight participants completed daily 3-min motor imagery homework, which consisted of rethinking the previous session's dance. The ad hoc pleasantness questionnaire, the Yale Global Tic Severity Scale (YGTSS) [19], and the Beck Depression Inventory—Second Edition (BDI-II) [20] are among the three tests. After taking YGTSS and BDI-II into account, sessions 1 and 7 for song 1 were compared, and sessions 2 and 8 for song 2. Song 2 demonstrated YGTSS improvements that were greater in the music group than in the control group. Music had an impact on the BDI-II scores [5].

## *1.2 Musicians, Singers, and Songwriters with Tourette Syndrome*

Several notable musicians have been associated with Tourette Syndrome (TS) throughout history, however, many of those links had to be made after the neurological illness was discovered. Several of these situations remain disputed because of a lack of understanding during the time when some of these individuals were alive.

Because TS is a comorbid disorder, it is frequently misdiagnosed as ADHD, Obsessive–Compulsive Disorder (OCD), and other impulse control problems. Beginning with Wolfgang Amadeus Mozart, one of the most inventive composers of all time. Erythema nodosum, sore throat, upper respiratory infections, acute post-infectious polyarthritis, and various additional ailments thought to be typhoid fever were among his childhood illnesses [22, 23]. He wrote almost 600 pieces and died in 1791, which was thought to be caused by acute rheumatic illness, although nothing has been proven [22]. Coprographia and coprolalia, as well as the excessive use of filthy vocabulary and vulgar language, were among the key signs that led others to believe Mozart had TS [24, 25]. In the mid- and late-twentieth century, Kurt Cobain was a brilliant singer and composer [26]. He experienced ADHD and OCD symptoms, such as collecting objects and documenting thoughts, throughout his childhood. The key symptom that prompted people to question his TS diagnosis was his involuntary ocular spasms at an early age [26]. Motor and vocal tics became obvious during interviews, but they worsened when he was upset or smoking. Other musicians diagnosed with Tourette Syndrome include Michael Wolff, Nick van Bloss, and James Durbin [26]. Many other musicians have been shown to exhibit different facial expressions, but unlike tics, there were no vocal actions. According to a study of twenty classical pianists, the players displayed facial emotions during the performance, including periods of tension, but not before or after [27]. Involuntary grimacing and facial tension are rarely mentioned because they don't appear to impair performance very often. Some artists have attempted to reinforce the expressions and use them as musical cues. Some claim that these expressions appeared when technical issues arose, but became habitual and continued [27, 28].

## 2 Internet of Things (IoT) and Mobile Health (mHealth), Music and TS

In a case study using wearable technology, Scataglini et al. [9] investigated the impact of rhythmic auditory stimulation on the modulation of tics in TS [10]. The procedure involved simultaneously recording images from a camera and synchronized tic detection recordings from a wearable device placed on the patient's trunk. Utilizing a five-level scale to characterize intensity and frequency, the Advene Software suite was used to integrate data from video and acceleration signals [10]. Music was played both at home and in a medical center, both with and without earphones and in and out of the examiner's presence. Results showed that auditory stimulation in a 4/4 beat reduced the frequency of intense tics. Particularly, listening to the same music using earbuds results in a 67% drop [10]. However, during COVID-19 pandemic telehealth ambulatory contacts rose significantly transforming health and care in telehealth and remote patient monitoring [28]. But patients don't always have wearables with them and may not want to use them because they are afraid to use them or don't want to buy them. Sending them wearables isn't always easy. This is because there is also a problem not only with hygiene but also with the ability to use them without an examiner. This is particularly difficult in Tourette Syndrome where the tics are motor involving extremes' lower and upper body but also the face. In this case, the accelerometry is not able to understand facial expressions (tics) of slight identity. Consequently, video recording can be adopted especially for facial tics.

## *2.1 A Telehealth Protocol*

To solve this, an online study with the possibility of being transformed into a telehealth service was tested into a health subject to see its ability to monitor tics without physically collaborating with the subjects. The entirety of the experiment was conducted online through Team web call meetings as well as using google forms for data collection.

Before the start of the experiment, the participant was asked to fill out a survey as a questionnaire and sign an informed consent. This questionnaire asked demographic information as well as music preferences (see Table 1).

The music was divided into four different categories: heavy metal, rap/hip-hop, pop, and classical. Each genre, such as serenity, joy, vitality, and rage, was intended to represent a particular emotion. The emotions, which included heightened, lowered, positive, and negative emotions, were selected from each range that was intended to be examined. For the duration of the experiment, one song from each musical genre was

**Table 1** A preliminary questionnaire

| | |
|---|---|
| 1 | Age |
| 2 | Gender |
| 3 | Body height, body mass |
| 4 | Do you like playing music? Yes/no, which instruments? |
| 5 | Which music do you like? |
| 6 | Which kind of music relaxes you? |
| 7 | Which kind of music makes you happy? |
| 8 | Do you prefer to listen the music at home, in which environment? |
| 9 | Do you use earphones or not? |
| 10 | Does the music create a beneficial effect? |
| 11 | How often do you listen to music? A day, a week? |
| 12 | Do you prefer classical, pop, rock, or heavy metal? Which one don't you like? |
| 13 | Does the music create a mental or physical rhythm or both? |
| 14 | Do you see a difference if you wear or do not wear earphones? |
| 15 | Which effect provokes the music on your body? |
| 16 | Do you like to be monitored or do you feel observed? And does this create stress for you? |

picked and played; the song was chosen based on its level of popularity at the outset of the study. The sole additional requirement for song selection was that all songs have a 4/4 time signature to improve uniformity and lessen the likelihood of unrelated elements. Online meeting recordings were made through Teams web calls, which were then used for visual assessments. The subject was instructed to stay in a quiet room with and without the earphones attached to a device, such as a smartphone, for the first part of the experiment in front of a Team Web call. Two views were captured: one full body in standing, and a second one asking the subject to sit putting her/his camera close-up of the head and shoulders. After a no-music test, the participant listened to 150 s of each musical style. The individual was asked to complete a brief survey after each of the five tests with and without wearing the earphones (no music, classical, pop, rap, and heavy metal) to assess how their tics were impacted and their present emotional condition. Successive tics were quantified using the Teams web call video recordings imported into Advene software, where it was possible to assign a level of intensity from 1 to 5 according to the previous study by Scataglini et al. [9, 10]. This protocol may be useful during the epidemic phase. Teleconsulting not only broadens the scope of Tourette syndrome assessment but also this permits the patient to be supervised by removing the "white coat" effect, which might result in the formation of further tics. The patient is placed in a comfortable setting where he/she is watched virtually. Furthermore, this approach may be useful for communication and patient monitoring prior to or during deep brain stimulation or pharmacotherapy. It also enables cost savings for both the medical center and the patient, who must travel to specialist centers following costly and stressful visits that are sometimes unpaid. Furthermore, this process may enable borderless teleconsultation services for both the doctor and the patient, serving as a comparison service between many specialists from different countries that do international research.

## 3 Conclusion

The purpose of this chapter was to provide an overview of the relationship between music, musicians, and Tourette Syndrome. Music has been shown to be beneficial for Tourette syndrome. This beneficial effect can be quantified using the mHealth and telehealth protocols presented. In the future, more research into how different aspects of music, as well as different types of musical activities, can contribute to TS research and help TS in everyday life, should be undertaken.

## References

1. Cravedi, E., Deniau, E., Giannitelli, M., Xavier, J., Hartmann, A., Cohen, D.: Tourette syndrome and other neurodevelopmental disorders: a comprehensive review. Child Adolesc. Psychiatry Ment. Health, **11**(1), (2017)

2. Powell, H., Kushner, H.I.: Mozart at play, in Music, Neurology, and Neuroscience: Historical Connections and Perspectives, pp. 277–291. Elsevier, (2015)
3. Scahill, L., et al.: Contemporary assessment and pharmacotherapy of Tourette syndrome. NeuroRx **3**(2), 192–206 (2006)
4. Bergin, A., Waranch, H.R., Brown, J., Carson, K., Singer, H.S.: Relaxation therapy in tourette syndrome: A pilot study. Pediatr. Neurol. **18**(2), 136–142 (1998)
5. Dina, Z., Rago, S., Cancer, A., Antonietti, A.: Music-dance-imaging training for young adults with Tourette Syndrome. Life Span Disabil. **23**, 187–209, 200AD
6. Brancatisano, O., Baird, A., Thompson, W.F.: Why is music therapeutic for neurological disorders? The Therapeutic Music Capacities Model. Neurosci. Biobehav. Rev. **112**, 600–615 (2020)
7. Page, S.J., Levine, P., Sisto, S.A., Johnston, M.V.: Mental practice combined with physical practice for upper-limb motor deficit in subacute stroke. Phys. Ther. **81**(8), 1455–1462 (2001)
8. Bodeck, S., Lappe, C., Evers, S.: Tic-reducing effects of music in patients with Tourette's syndrome: Self-reported and objective analysis. J. Neurol. Sci. **352**(1–2), 41–47 (2015)
9. Scataglini, S., Fusca, M., Andreoni, G., Porta, M.: "Application of wearable monitoring system in tourette syndrome assessment." Lecture Notes of the Institute for Computer Sciences, pp. 100–106. Springer International Publishing, Social Informatics and Telecommunications Engineering, Cham (2017)
10. Scataglini, S.: Effect of rhythmic music auditory stimulation on tics modulation in tourette syndrome: A case study. Open access j. neurol. neurosurg., **5**(5), (2017)
11. Goetz, C.G., Pappert, E.J., Louis, E.D., Raman, R., Leurgans, S.: Advantages of a modified scoring method for the Rush Video-Based Tic Rating Scale. Mov. Disord. **14**(3), 502–506 (1999)
12. Thaut, M. H., Rice, R.R., Braun Janzen, T., Hurt-Thaut, C., Mcintosh, G.C.: Rhythmic auditory stimulation for reduction of falls in Parkinson'sdisease: a randomized controlled study. Clin Rehabil, **33**(1), 34–43(2019)
13. Pohl, P., Dizdar, N., Hallert, E.: The ronnie gardiner rhythm and music method—a feasibility study in Parkinson's disease. Disabil. Rehabil. **35**(26), 2197–2204 (2013)
14. Trimble, M., Hesdorffer, D.: Music and the brain: the neuroscience of music and musical appreciation. BJPsych Int. **14**(2), 28–31 (2017)
15. Colautti, L., Magenes, S., Rago, S., Zanaboni Dina, C., Alice Cancer, Antonietti, A.: Creative thinking in tourette's syndrome: An uncharted topic. Front. Psychol., **12**, (2021)
16. Chan, S.-Y., Chen, C.-F.: Effects of an active music therapy program on functional fitness in community older adults. J. Nurs. Res. **28**(5), e111 (2020)
17. Wikipedia contributors, "Gioca jouer," Wikipedia, The Free Encyclopedia. [Online].Available: https://it.wikipedia.org/w/index.php?title=Gioca_jouer&oldid=128350593.
18. Wikipedia contributors.: Don Lurio," Wikipedia, The Free Encyclopedia. (2022). [Online].Available https://en.wikipedia.org/w/index.php?title=Don_Lurio&oldid=1103163964
19. Haas, M. et al.: Yale global tic severity scale (YGTSS): Psychometric quality of the gold standard for tic assessment based on the large-scale EMTICS study. Front. Psychiatry, **12**, (2021)
20. Beck, A.T., Steer, R.A., Brown, G.K.: Manual for the beck depression inventory-II. Psychological Corporation, San Antonio, TX (1996)
21. Monaco, F., Servo, S., Cavanna, A.E.: Famous people with Gilles de la Tourette syndrome? J. Psychosom. Res. **67**(6), 485–490 (2009)
22. Karhausen, L.R.: Weeding Mozart's medical history. J. R. Soc. Med. **91**(10), 546–550 (1998)
23. Bhattacharyya, K., Rai, S.: Famous people with Tourette's syndrome: Dr. Samuel Johnson (yes) & Wolfgang Amadeus Mozart (may be): Victims of Tourette′s syndrome? Ann. Indian Acad. Neurol., **18**(2), 157 (2015)
24. Aterman, K.: Did Mozart have tourette's syndrome?: Some comments on Mozart's language. Perspect. Biol. Med. **37**(2), 247–258 (1994)

25. Kammer, T.: Mozart in the neurological department—who has the tic?. In: Neurological Disorders in Famous Artists—Part 2 (pp. 184–192). KARGER, Basel (2007)
26. Camargo, C.H.F., Bronzini, A.: Tourette's syndrome in famous musicians. Arq. Neuropsiquiatr. **73**(12), 1038–1040 (2015)
27. Lees, A.J., Swash, M.: Face-making: task-specific facial tensions and grimacing in musicians. J. Neurol. Neurosurg. Psychiatry **90**(10), 1180–1182 (2019)
28. Jankovic, J., Ashoori, A.: Movement disorders in musicians: Movement Disorders in Musicians. Mov. Disord. **23**(14), 1957–1965 (2008)
29. Weiner, J.P., Bandeian, S., Hatef, E., Lans, D., Liu, A., Lemke, K.W.: In-person and telehealth ambulatory contacts and costs in a large US insured cohort before and during the COVID-19 pandemic. JAMA Netw. Open **4**(3), e212618 (2021)

# Artificial Intelligence Applications and Social Assistive Robotics to Counteract Cognitive Decline in the Older Population: Evidence from Trials in Real Settings

**R. Bevilacqua, A. Margaritini, G. Cucchieri, C. Giammarchi, G. Amabili, and E. Maranesi**

## 1 Introduction

Currently, there are a plethora of SARs aimed at promoting physical and cognitive health and prolonging the older person's independence. Indeed, with advancing age, difficulties come into play in several domains, from physical to cognitive, such as memory, attention, language, and all executive functions [1]. This decline, both physical and cognitive, that the older person undergoes inevitably, leads to difficulties and limitations, even in the simplest, but most basic, daily activities, such as eating, dressing, and washing. In addition to this, a common risk faced by the older people is that of falls, which can lead to further physical limitations or hospitalization [2]. As a consequence, the lowering of mood, the onset of anxiety problems, and feelings

R. Bevilacqua · A. Margaritini · G. Cucchieri · C. Giammarchi · G. Amabili (✉) · E. Maranesi
IRCCS INRCA, Scientific Direction, Ancona, Italy
e-mail: g.amabili@inrca.it

R. Bevilacqua
e-mail: r.bevilacqua@inrca.it

A. Margaritini
e-mail: a.margaritini2@inrca.it

G. Cucchieri
e-mail: g.cucchieri@inrca.it

C. Giammarchi
e-mail: c.giammarchi@inrca.it

E. Maranesi
e-mail: e.maranesi@inrca.it

 
S. Scataglini et al. (eds.), *mHealth and Human-Centered Design Towards Enhanced Health, Care, and Well-Being*, Studies in Big Data 120,
https://doi.org/10.1007/978-981-99-3989-3_9

of loneliness and worthlessness [3], which further worsen the cognitive state, are somehow expected, causing the person to enter a vicious cycle.

It is therefore evident the increasing need to support not only physical, but also emotional and cognitive maintenance of the older population, which are considered factors that influence each other, from a biopsychosocial perspective [4]. To prevent cognitive decline, it is essential that older adults have meaningful and stable relationships, stay as active as possible, and play a role within society [5, 6].

As in recent years there has been a growing shortage of healthcare workers, which, combined with the increased rate of older population, makes the search for innovative solutions of utmost importance [7], the implementation of SARs offers a viable solution for providing interventions aimed at preventing the decline in a person's cognitive and functional abilities [8]. In fact, by including them into the older person's daily routine, it is possible to manage the assessment and the monitoring of the cognitive functions, to collect information on the disease's progression, and to guarantee the adherence to physical and cognitive exercise protocols [9]. Moreover, the introduction of SARs may help to prevent burnout phenomena in caregivers and family members while ensuring that the older people receive the right amount and quality of care.

Despite this, the uptake of such technologies seems to be far from being widespread [10, 11] although research suggests a beneficial effect of their use with cognitive function [12–14]. In fact, SARs seems to be still in its beginning stages [15] and they are not yet adopted in daily practice, but only at experimental and research level [16]. Moreover, most of the studies have been focused on overcoming physical disabilities and mobility limitations, leaving out cognitive functions [2].

One reason for this, of course, is the difficulty in determining precisely the positive role of those solutions, by adopting an evidence-based approach. Indeed, the use of social robots for supporting cognitive decline has shown results that are not always linear and consistent [17]. Especially in terms of anxiety, agitation, depression, the benefits of social robots are not always significant [18, 19]. In addition, when dealing with a heterogeneous population as the older one, especially in terms of cognitive support, it is vital to consider several variables that may affect the adoption of SARs such as [20]: overall health status and motivation, level of cognitive functioning at the time of the first assessment, and the emotional-psychological state [21, 22].

As it is well known that the elderly's acceptance of a robot is a fundamental step to guarantee its adoption and continued use [23], the deep understanding of the cognitive decline, in terms of causes and consequences, is needed first and foremost for a good design phase. However, many published studies were focused on a more design oriented approach, to collect information to support ergonomics and usability of SARs [24, 25], but failing to fully understand how to properly include the cognitive needs in the developmental process.

The paper aims to update the knowledge on the efficacy and applicability of social robotics in the context of supporting cognitive decline in the older population, from prevention and self-management of initial cognitive impairments to the most advanced phases of dementia. The analysis conducted should be a starting point for health professionals but also policymakers and health providers to understand how to properly introduce SARs in multicomponent interventions, dedicated to the older population affected by cognitive decline at every stage. Interventions that targeted several domains of health and psychological well-being in older adults, in fact, have been found as promising solutions to address the needs of the older population in a holistic way [26], and they can be easily supported through technology. In particular, SARs may play a key role in supporting the psychological and social connectedness needs, in addition to coaching the older people in remaining active and self-managing their cognitive difficulties as long as possible.

# 2 Methods

## 2.1 Literature Search and Study Selection

The literature was reviewed in May 2022. In order to explore the latest works in social robotics, the data were collected by analyzing manuscripts and articles published in the last 10 years (from May 2012 to May 2022) on PubMed, Scopus, and Elsevier databases. Based on internal discussion with the multidisciplinary team, papers addressing the efficacy of the SARs to support the cognitive status of the older population were searched by entering the following keywords, and the combinations thereof: social robot, cognitive decline, dementia, mild cognitive impairment, old*, artificial intelligence. Within the preliminary search, 146 articles were identified from PubMed, 125 from Scopus, and 4298 from Elsevier. The findings were analyzed and screened by 3 experts of the team: a bioengineer, a clinical psychologist, and an electronic engineer. First, the results were screened by analyzing the title and the abstract, as well as looking for deduplication of the findings. A further researcher confirmed the accuracy of the selection and screened for any possible omission. Once went through the aforementioned steps, 67 articles were identified: 21 from PubMed, 31 from Scopus, and 15 from Elsevier.

The overall objective of the analysis is to provide a clear understanding of the state of the art in the field of social robotics for dementia care and cognitive decline support. In particular, the achievement of knowledge on the efficacy and applicability of social robotics in specific contexts of use, from prevention and self-management to dementia care, will allow the faster adoption and uptake of SARs.

## 2.2 Selection Strategy

We included any type of clinical trials, such as Randomized Controlled Trials (RCTs) or before-and-after study, written in English, and focused on the use of SARs for supporting the older people's cognitive status. Thus, we selected studies meeting the criteria below

1. Studies conducted on adult aged $\geq$65 years.
2. Studies with the aim of examining the efficacy of the newest applications in the field of SARs for older adults.
3. Any type of clinical trials.
4. Before-after comparison of a single group, and comparison between groups.

On the contrary, we excluded studies that met the following criteria:

1. Conference proceedings.
2. Studies for which the full text was not found.
3. Studies written in languages other than English.
4. Technical papers.
5. Qualitative studies.
6. Review articles.

Review articles were excluded, but already included in the dissertation.

### *2.3 Data Collection*

After applying the inclusion/exclusion criteria on the full text articles, 13 studies were selected: 10 from PubMed, 3 from Scopus, and 0 from Elsevier database. Figure 1 shows the flowchart search strategy applied.

## 3 Results

### *3.1 General Characteristics of the Study Population*

A total of 13 papers were included [27–39]. All the studies were about older people with a mean age of 83.3 ($\pm$8.2) years. The number of participants involved in all the studies is 1540, ranging from 10 to 455. From the information obtained from some articles [27, 29–39], there were 417 males and 1099 females. The participants considered were affected by either dementia [27–36, 39] or mild cognitive impairments [37, 38]. Moreover, the robots tested are of two types: pet robots [27–35] and humanoid robots [36–39]. Table 1 describes the SARs tested in the interventions, while the taxonomy of the main findings from the study selection is available in Fig. 2.

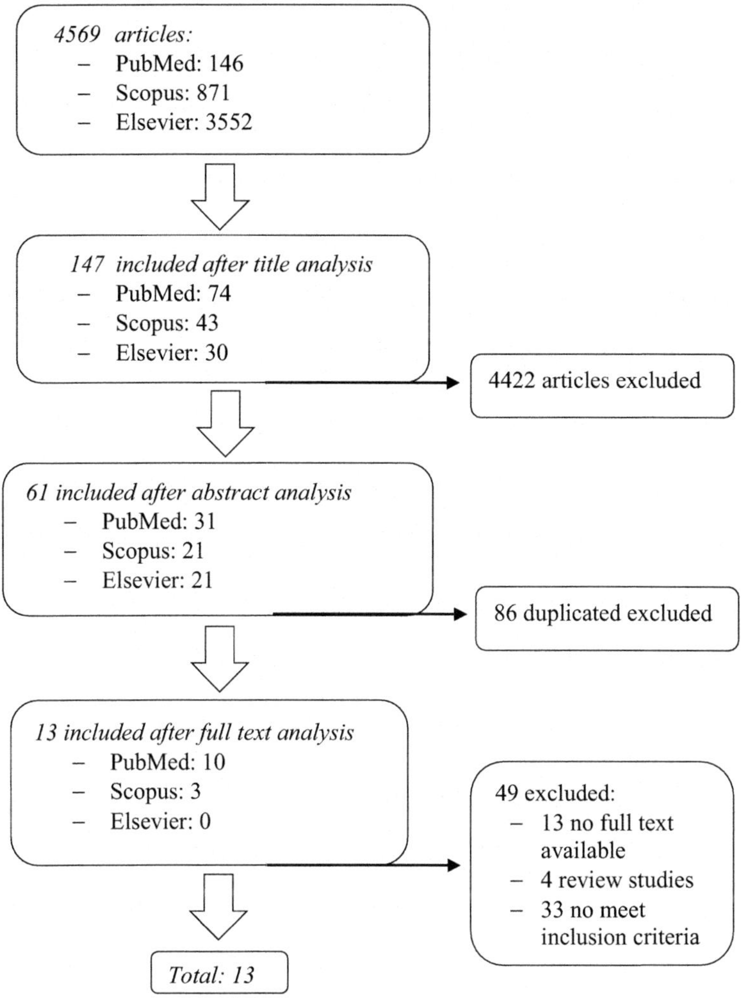


**Fig. 1** Flowchart of the search strategy applied

## *3.2 Descriptive Analysis and Outcome Measures*

In this section the results of selected studies are described, whereas Table 2 shows the author, the year, and the country of the studies, the enrolled population, the SAR used, the protocol, and the measurements. From the literature review, it is evident that in patients with dementia, there is a tendency to use Paro [27–35], the baby harp seal that is an advanced, interactive therapeutic robot. PARO was initially developed to bring psychological relief and joy to persons with dementia. These studies aimed to investigate the effect of Paro on symptoms such as anxiety and agitation, as well as quality of life, social interaction, facial expressiveness, motor activity, and sleep

**Table 1** Description of SARs tested in selected interventions

| Social assistive robot | Characteristics |
|---|---|
| 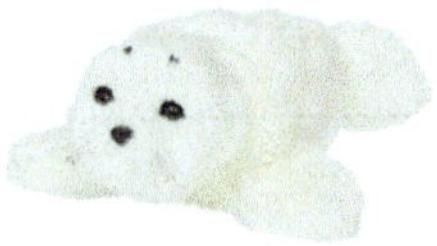 | PARO is a baby seal, covered in soft fur, under which sensors and actuators are hidden. PARO senses the user's caresses and reacts with more or less pleasant sounds and movements, depending on the gentleness or violence with which it is treated |
| 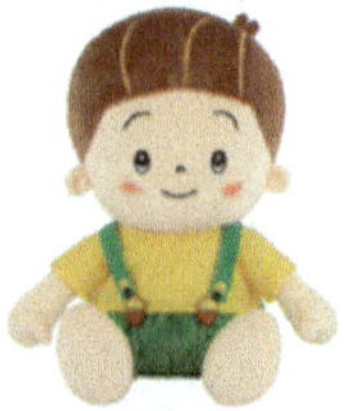 | Kabochan is a soft robot dressed as a pumpkin, 28 cm tall, that interacts affectively with older adults. It is able to speak, sing, and nod gracefully in response to its owner's touch and words, sensed by the five sensors placed on its mouth, head, and hands. In addition, Kabochan offers interactive games, including pose play, flag play, and vocal singing exercises |
| 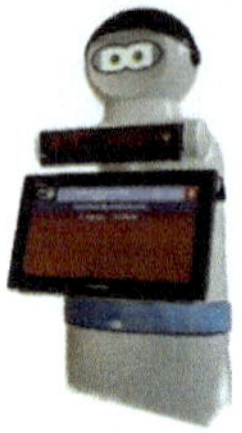 | MARIO is a humanoid social robot, 1.5 m tall and equipped with a tablet. The tablet offers various applications, including playing songs, reading news, playing cognitive games, and showing pictures. MARIO, which is equipped with a microphone, is capable of illustrating these activities (reading, singing) but not conversing with the user |
| 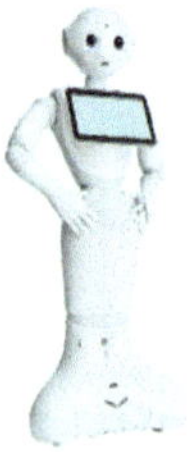 | Pepper is a humanoid robot another 1.20 m, equipped with a touch screen at chest height and wheels that allow it to move in vast spaces. With its touch sensors, microphone, LED eye illumination, video camera, touch screen and speaker Pepper manages to provide excellent user interaction. Pepper is one of the most advanced social robots precisely in terms of HRI: the mobility of its upper limbs, hands, and head confer a high level of expressiveness |
| 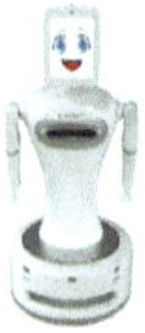 | Sil-bot is a 1.14-m-tall humanoid robot equipped with wheels and an autonomous driving system. Interaction can be by voice or tablet, and Sil-bot can also recognize the user's emotions by analyzing the user's gaze. Features include cognitive games and reminder activity |

partners. In these study cases, the protocol was the same: older people with dementia participated in group or individual unstructured activities with Paro that lasted an average of 30 min, 2–3 times a week. In particular, Moyle et al. [31] showed how older people with dementia who used Paro for 10 weeks instead of a plush toy were more verbally and visually engaged, and their pleasure was improved as well. The

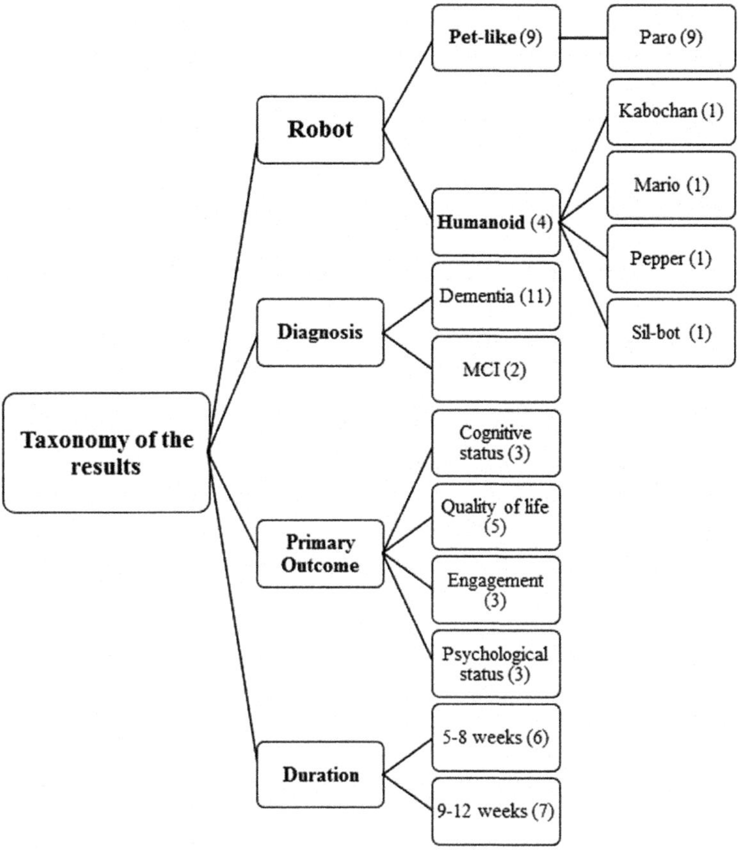


**Fig. 2** Taxonomy of the main findings from selected study

impact of PARO in interactive terms is showed also by Kelly et al. [32], who reported an increase in speaking and petting interactions. One of the greatest benefits of PARO is the reduction of agitation and stress, as well as decreasing daytime and nighttime step count [34], and observed pain [33]. Moyle et al. [34] also reported a decrease in nighttime physical activity. In line with the aforementioned studies, Pu et al. [36] found that after the first week PARO impacted on increasing the night sleep period, and after the sixth week also on decreasing the daytime sleep causing an increase of the daytime wakefulness. These results underline Paro's effectiveness in managing different moods and agitation, and can be correlated to reduction of medications. In fact, Jøranson et al. [27] administered Paro twice a week for 30 min to older people with dementia with symptoms of agitation and depression living in nursing homes. According to this study, Paro seems to be a suitable non-pharmacological treatment for neuropsychiatric symptoms and should be considered as a useful tool in clinical practice, since the experimental group used significantly less psychotropic medication compared with the control group after the end of intervention. Moreover, the same research group investigated the effects of Paro on quality of life in the same kind of patients [29]. Authors state how the use of Paro in patients with severe dementia declines typical symptoms such as agitation and depression, as well as improves their engagement, often challenged by apathy and withdrawal.

With regard to all aspects involving behavior, affectivity, and social interaction, respectively measured by Liang et al. [28] with facial expressions and communication with the staff. This study showed highlighted as individuals with greater cognitive functioning were more responsive to Paro, thus emphasizes the importance of developing personalized and effective ways to improve the well-being of people with dementia, using technological devices.

Only one paper [32] analyzes the use of Paro in hospitalized patients with dementia, in order to determine physiological effects and describe social-affective interactions. In this case, the differences in pre- and post-physiological measures were not clinically significant but participants demonstrated benefits with Paro interactions in terms of gesturing, speaking, and moving.

With respect to previous studies, Jones et al. [30] presented conflicting findings. The study associated severe agitation with poor effectiveness of PARO, since older people with higher levels of agitation worsened after the intervention. However, people with lower agitation and higher cognitive capabilities responded better to the trial.

Regarding studies using humanoid robots, not the same robot was used but different robots such as Kabochan [36], Mario [39], Pepper [38], or Sil-Bot [37], in older patients with dementia [36, 39] or mild cognitive impairment [37, 38].

In particular, Kabochan, a humanoid companion robot with appearance, voice and motions resembling a 3-years old boy, was used to test the reduction of dementia symptoms. Unfortunately, this study found no significant improvements in cognitive function or quality of life for participants.

Whelan et al. [39] instead, investigated how Mario, a humanoid social robot, affects the resilience of people with dementia. The findings revealed that this population required skilled facilitation to use Mario. Moreover, sessions with Mario increased the well-being of patients by providing a meaningful activity that reinforced their positive self-concept.

However, in the case of patients with mild cognitive impairment, the protocols involved humanoid robot-supported cognitive training.

In Manca et al. [38], a music-based memory game has been played with the humanoid robot Pepper. In this context, the robot was received with more enthusiasm by the older adults, thus improving their level of engagement.

In Park et al. [37], the humanoid robot Sil-Bot has been used in order to improve cognitive function and depression decline in older adults with mild cognitive impairment. During the experimentation, the participants were guided to solve problems or performed a physical, musical, or art activity while the robot displayed around 30 emotional expressions to compliment and encourage the patients. At the end of training, participants had significantly greater improvement in cognitive function, memory, depression, and executive function.

**Table 2** Descriptive analysis of the included clinical studies

| Study, year | Population | | Intervention | Robot | Measurements |
|---|---|---|---|---|---|
| | Participants in experimental group (EG) | Participants in control group (CG) | | | |
| Jøranson et al. 2016 [27] | $n = 27$ older adults with dementia (19 F/8 M)<br>Age: 83.9 ± 7.2 years | $n = 26$ older adults with dementia (18 F/8 M)<br>Age: 84.1 ± 6.7 years | 24 sessions of 30 min each interacting with Paro; frequency: twice a week over 12 weeks<br>Follow-up: 3 months | Paro | Quality of Life in Late-Stage Dementia scale |
| Liang et al. 2017 [28] | $n = 13$ older adults with dementia (8 F/5 M)<br>Age range; 67–98 years | $n = 11$ older adults with dementia (7 F/4 M)<br>Age range; 67–98 years | 30-min unstructured group sessions with Paro at the day care center (2–3 times a week for 6 weeks) + taking Paro at home for all the 6 weeks | Paro | Primary outcome: observations of the care recipients' behavior, affect, and social responses were recorded using a time sampling method<br>Observations of interactions with Paro for participants in the intervention were also recorded |
| Jøranson et al. 2015 [29] | $n = 27$ older adults with dementia (19 F/8 M)<br>Age: 83.9 ± 7.2 years | $n = 26$ older adults with dementia (18 F/8 M)<br>Age: 84.1 ± 6.7 years | 24 group sessions with Paro (max. 6 people per group) for 30 min;<br>Frequency: twice a week for 12 weeks<br>Follow-up: 3 months | Paro | Brief Agitation Rating Scale (BARS)<br>Cornell Scale for Symptoms of Depression in Dementia (CSDD) |
| Jones et al. 2018 [30] | $n = 138$ older adults with dementia (101 F/37 M)<br>Age: 84 ± 8.4 years | – | 30 individual, non-facilitated, 15-min sessions with PARO; frequency: 3 times a week for 10 weeks | Paro | Primary outcomes: Participants' levels of engagement, mood states, and agitation at week 10, assessed by video observation and Cohen-Mansfield Agitation Inventory-Short Form (CMAI-SF) |

(continued)

**Table 2** (continued)

| Study, year | Population | | Intervention | Robot | Measurements |
|---|---|---|---|---|---|
| | Participants in experimental group (EG) | Participants in control group (CG) | | | |
| Moyle et al. 2017 [31] | Paro group: $n = 138$ older adults with dementia (101 F/37 M)<br>Age: 84 ± 8.4 years | Plush Toy group: $n = 140$ older adults with dementia (114 F/26 M)<br>Age: 86 ± 7.6 years<br>Usual Care group: $n = 137$ older adults with dementia (99 F/38 M)<br>Age: 85 ± 7.1 years | 30 individual, non-facilitated, 15-min session with PARO; frequency: 3 times a week for 10 weeks | Paro | Primary outcomes: changes in levels of engagement, mood states, and agitation after a 10-week intervention, and<br>Cohen-Mansfield Agitation Inventory Short Form<br>Secondary outcomes: short-term effects of the intervention for engagement, mood states, and agitation at weeks 1 and 5, as well as longer-term sustained effects post-intervention (week 15) for mood states and agitation |
| Kelly et al. 2020 [32] | $n = 55$ hospitalized older adults with dementia (38 F/17 M)<br>Age: 85.5 ± 8.1 years | - | 15-min with the Paro placed on the participant's lap or on the bedside stand in front of the participant; frequency: 2–3 times a week over 5–12 weeks | Paro | Primary outcomes: Delirium assessment (four-question Short CAM)<br>Physiologic measures (blood pressure, heart rate, respirations, oxygen saturation, stress, and pain levels)<br>Social and affective interaction measures |

(continued)

**Table 2** (continued)

| Study, year | Population | | Intervention | Robot | Measurements |
|---|---|---|---|---|---|
| | Participants in experimental group (EG) | Participants in control group (CG) | | | |
| Pu et al. 2020 [33] | $n = 21$ older adults with dementia (18 F/3 M)<br>Age: 86.48 ± 8.81 years | $n = 22$ older adults with dementia (18 F/3 M)<br>Age: 85.55 ± 5.80 years | 30 individual non-facilitated Paro-activity conducted for 30 min; frequency: 5 times a week for 6 weeks | Paro | Primary outcome: observational pain behaviors before and after each session. Secondary outcomes: pain level, agitation, depression, and anxiety measured at baseline and the end of week 6 |
| Moyle et al. 2018 [34] | Daytime | | 30 individual, non-facilitated, 15-min sessions with PARO; frequency: 3 times per week for 10 weeks | Paro | Changes in day- and nighttime motor activity and sleep after the 10-week intervention, during two single intervention days in weeks 5 and 10 respectively, and post-intervention (week 15) |
| | Paro group: $n = 67$ older adults with dementia (53 F/14 M)<br>Age: 84 ± 8.8 years | Plush Toy group: $n = 55$ older adults with dementia (42 F/13 M)<br>Age: 86 ± 7.6 years<br>Usual Care group: $n = 53$ older adults with dementia (35 F/18 M)<br>Age: 85 ± 6.9 years | | | |
| | Nighttime | | | | |

(continued)

**Table 2** (continued)

| Study, year | Population | | Intervention | Robot | Measurements |
|---|---|---|---|---|---|
| | Participants in experimental group (EG) | Participants in control group (CG) | | | |
| | Paro group: $n = 98$ older adults with dementia (76 F/22 M)<br>Age: 84 ± 8.4 years | Plush Toy group: $n = 95$ older adults with dementia (76 F/19 M)<br>Age: 87 ± 7.0 years<br>Usual Care group: $n = 87$ older adults with dementia (58 F/29 M)<br>Age: 85 ± 7.1 years | | | |
| Pu et al. 2020 [35] | $n = 21$ older adults with dementia and chronic pain (18 F/3 M)<br>Age: 86.48 ± 8.81 years | $n = 20$ older adults with dementia and chronic pain (11 F/9 M)<br>Age: 85.5 ± 6.02 years | 30-min social robot (Paro) condition; frequency: everyday for 6 weeks | Paro | Sleep and motor activity |
| Chen et al. 2020 [36] | $n = 52$ older adults with dementia (40 F/12 M)<br>Age: 87 ± 8.2 years | $n = 51$ older adults with dementia (42 F/9 M)<br>Age: 87.3 ± 6.6 years | The intervention consisted of 4 consecutive phases. Each phase lasted for 8 weeks. Kabochan was introduced in a non-facilitated, individual approach with EG for 8 weeks, then removed for 8 weeks, and then reintroduced for another 8 weeks. The control group received the usual standardized care | Kabochan | Primary outcomes: Neuropsychiatric Inventory Questionnaire Geriatric Depression Scale<br>Secondary outcomes: Hong Kong Montreal Cognitive Assessment 5-min Protocol<br>Modified Barthel Index for Activities of Daily Living Quality of Life-Alzheimer's disease scale |

(continued)

**Table 2** (continued)

| Study, year | Population | | Intervention | Robot | Measurements |
|---|---|---|---|---|---|
| | Participants in experimental group (EG) | Participants in control group (CG) | | | |
| Park et al. 2021 [37] | Robot group: $n = 45$ older adults with mild cognitive impairment (32 F/13 M)<br>Age: $75.5 \pm 5.9$ years | Traditional group: $n = 45$ older adults with mild cognitive impairment (23 F/22 M)<br>Age: $76.7 \pm 5.9$ years<br>No intervention group: $n = 45$ older adults with mild cognitive impairment (27 F/18 M)<br>Age: $75.6 \pm 6.6$ years | The training for robot and traditional groups consisted of a daily 60 min session, twice a week for six weeks | Robot Sil-Bot | Primary outcomes: Cognition (Mini-Mental State Examination-Dementia Screening)<br>Subjective Memory Complaints<br>Neuropsychological assessment (Consortium to Establish a Registry for Alzheimer's Disease, CERAD) |
| Manca et al. 2021 [38] | $n = 14$ older adults with mild cognitive impairments (9 F/5 M), divided into two groups associated with the two conditions considered in the test: "pepper" versus "tablet."<br>Age: $75.3 \pm 4.5$ years | | The experiment was organized in two different stages: (1) familiarizing with the humanoid robot Pepper and the tablet; (2) playing the music game with the humanoid robot and the tablet<br>The game was played two days a week with a total of 12 sessions over a month | Pepper | Outcomes: number of correct answers, wrong answers, number of answers not provided within the time limit, the time needed to complete the whole game, the time needed to respond to each answer, and the number of trials needed to provide 12 correct answers<br>User engagement<br>User's feedback |
| Whelan et al. 2020 [39] | $n = 10$ older adults with dementia (7 F/3 M)<br>Age: $83 \pm 10.1$ years | – | MARIO was offered to participants with dementia for up to 12 individual sessions, 3 times a week, during 5 weeks | Mario | Quality of Life in Alzheimer's disease The Resilience Scale |

# 4 Discussion

Recent evidence has shown that older people seem to prefer the interaction with robots than other technologies such as tablets to taking care of their own well-being [38], since the engagement is higher. Therefore, there are several robots that have been developed nowadays to counteract the symptoms of cognitive decline and to offer support to usual care, often affected by the shortage of personnel. Many social robots, especially pet-like, have been tested with people with dementia and mild cognitive impairment in order to understand how much they can help in this scenario, especially PARO seems to be the most used in dementia care [40, 41]. All the studies reported in this work evaluated the effect of using a social robot with respect to a control group, in order to measure the efficacy of the intervention. The most tested device is Paro, a seal robot designed to interact with people affected by moderate or mild cognitive impairment and dementia. Since the interaction with Paro mainly consists of tactile feedback, sounds, and small movements, resulting in a simulated pet-therapy, it seems to be preferably suitable for older people affected by dementia even in the moderate stage. In most studies [27–32, 34], the usage protocols established a 15–30 min' session, to be repeated 2–3 times per week, whereas in two studies [33, 35] the older people interacted with Paro for at least 5 days per week. On the assessment side, all the nine studies on Paro have shown at least one significant outcome in relation to its use, even though each study investigated slightly different dimensions. In particular, the interaction with Paro has been found to be effective in reducing agitation [29], especially in people with lower levels of anxiety at the beginning of the study [30], including both older people with dementia or with Mild Cognitive Impairment (MCI). Moreover, an improvement of the quality of sleep of the older users has been observed after some weeks of use in two studies, consisting in the reduction of daytime sleep in favor of an increase in the night time sleep and the reduction of physical activity during the night [34, 35]. Together with the overall improvement of the older people's quality of life [27], the use of Paro concurred also in reducing the psychotropic medications intake [27], the depression levels [29], and the observed pain [33]. Finally, the positive effects of the interaction with Paro have also resulted in a higher degree of engagement, improved communication, and enjoyment in daily life [28, 31–33]. Given the results achieved in the aforementioned studies, it can be said that Paro could offer a great support to usual care and professionals, thanks also to its limited cost, the simplicity in use and the short duration of the daily session. Concerning the older users with MCI, humanoid robots were found as most suited for them instead, since they are supposed to interact more actively. For this purpose, in fact, humanoid robots are designed to stimulate cognitive skills through games and other engaging tasks. By performing these activities in cooperation with the robot, the older users can reinforce their positive self-efficacy, as in the case of a study with MARIO [39]. Finally, Park et al. [37] found that interacting with humanoid robots may have a positive impact on cognitive status, executive function, and depression. Even though several studies demonstrate the beneficial effects of introducing pet-like and human-like robots in the treatment of people with cognitive impairment or dementia, some evidence has shown controversial results. In some studies [30, 33], no significant reduction in anxiety and agitation was found, whereas in the study of Park et al. the older participants who underwent traditional therapy have shown a greater improvement in memory and executive functions with respect to the participants who underwent the robotic intervention with a humanoid robot, the Sil-Bot. Other two studies did not find any improvement on health and physiological measures after the interaction with Paro [32] and Kabochan [36]. Moreover, the lack of evidence about long-term effects of robotic therapy and the lead back to the worsening of neuropsychiatric symptoms once the intervention is suspended [36], may represent relevant barriers to the spread of social robots in the clinical sector.

## 5 Summary/Conclusion

Even if there a plethora of useful studies in this field, the uptake of SARs in dementia care is still limited. This review would like to inform future psychosocial interventions that can favor from the introduction of SARs in dementia care settings and support to cognitive decline. By understanding the characteristics and effectiveness of these technological solutions, health professionals, policymakers, and health providers may understand how to properly introduce SARs at every stage of cognitive decline. In particular, SARs may play a key role in supporting the psychological and social connectedness needs, in addition to coaching the older people in remaining active and self-managing their cognitive difficulties as long as possible. The promising results of existing studies should encourage investigating and testing the potentiality of social robotics for the older population, to counteract societal issue, like the shortage of health caregivers, for example, as well as clinical issue, as the increasing need of cognitive support to allow the older people to stay active and be part of the community. In order to increase the knowledge on the long-term efficacy of social robots in assisting the older people with MCI or dementia, it is necessary to extend the duration of the trials, especially those one in real settings.

## References

1. Van Patten, R., Keller, A.V., Maye, J.E., Jeste, D.V., Depp, C., Riek, L.D., Twamley, E.W.: Home-based cognitively assistive robots: maximizing cognitive functioning and maintaining independence in older adults without dementia. Clin. Interv. Aging. **15**, 1129–1139 (2020)
2. Ganesan, B., Gowda, T., Al-Jumaily, A., Fong, K.N.K., Meena, S.K., Tong, R.K.Y.: Ambient assisted living technologies for older adults with cognitive and physical impairments: a review. Eur. Rev. Med. Pharmacol. Sci. **23**(23), 10470–10481 (2019)
3. Ang, G.C., Low, S.L., How, C.H.: Approach to falls among the elderly in the community. Singap. Med. J. **61**(3), 116–121 (2020)
4. Miles, E.: Biopsychosocial model. In: Gellman, M.D., Turner, J.R. (eds.) Encyclopedia of Behavioral Medicine. Springer, New York, NY (2013)

5. Dodge, H.H., Zhu, J., Mattek, N., Bowman, M., Ybarra, O., Wild, K., Loewenstein, D.A., Kaye, J.A.: Web-enabled Conversational Interactions as a Means to Improve Cognitive Functions: Results of a 6-Week Randomized Controlled Trial. Alzheimer's & Dementia (New York, N. Y.), vol. 1(1), pp. 1–12 (2015)
6. Krueger, K.R., Wilson, R.S., Kamenetsky, J.M., Barnes, L.L., Bienias, J.L., Bennett, D.A.: Social engagement and cognitive function in old age. Exp. Aging Res. **35**, 45–60 (2009)
7. England, K., Alcorn, C.: Growing care gaps, shrinking state? Home care workers and the fair labor standards act. Camb. J. Reg. Econ. Soc. **11**, 443–457 (2018)
8. Mitzner, T.L., Chen, T.L., Kemp, C.C., Rogers, W.A.: Identifying the potential for robotics to assist older adults in different living environments. Int. J. Soc. Robot. **6**(2), 213–227 (2014)
9. Mancioppi, G., Fiorini, L., Timpano, S.M., Cavallo, F.: Novel technological solutions for assessment, treatment, and assistance in mild cognitive impairment. Front. Neuroinform. **13**, 58 (2019)
10. Robinson, H., MacDonald, B., Broadbent, E.: The role of healthcare robots for older people at home: a review. Int. J. Soc. Robot. **6**(4), 575–591 (2014)
11. Alnajjar, F., Khalid, S., Vogan, A.A., Shimoda, S., Nouchi, R., Kawashima, R.: Emerging cognitive intervention technologies to meet the needs of an aging population: a systematic review. Front. Aging Neurosci. **11**, 291 (2019)
12. Yaghoubzadeh, R., Kopp, S.: Enabling robust and fluid spoken dialogue with cognitively impaired users. In: Proceedings of the 18th Annual SIGdial Meeting on Discourse and Dialogue (Saarbrücken, Germany: Association for Computational Linguistics), pp. 273–283 (2017)
13. Otake-Matsuura, M., Tokunaga, S., Watanabe, K., Abe, M.S., Sekiguchi, T., Sugimoto, H., et al.: Cognitive intervention through photo-integrated conversation moderated by robots (PICMOR) program: a randomized controlled trial. Front. Robot. AI **8** (2021)
14. Van Patten, R., Keller, A.V., Maye, J.E., Jeste, D.V., Depp, C., Riek, L.D., et al.: Home based cognitively assistive robots: maximizing cognitive functioning and maintaining independence in older adults without dementia. Clin. Interv. Aging. **15**, 1129–1139 (2020)
15. Luperto, M., Monroy, J., Renoux, J., Lunardini, F., Basilico, N., Bulgheron, M., Cangelosi, A., Cesari, M., Cid, M., Ianes, A., Gonzalez-Jimenez, J., Kounoudes, A., Mari, D., Prisacariu, V., Savanovic, A., Ferrant, S., Borghes, N.A.: Integration of social welfare robots, IoT, virtual communities, and smart objects to assist elderly people living independently at home: the MoveCare project. Int. J. Soc. Robot., 1–31 (2022)
16. Fischinger, D., Einramhof, P., Papoutsakis, K., et al.: Hobbit, a care robot supporting independent living at home: first prototype and lessons learned. Robot. Auton. Syst. **75**, 60–78 (2016)
17. Tokunaga, S., Tamura, K.,Otake-Matsuura, M.A.: Dialogue-based system with photo and storytelling for older adults: toward daily cognitive training. Front. Robot. AI **8**, 644964 (2021)
18. Abbott, R., Orr, N., McGill, P., et al.: How do "robopets" impact the health and well-being of residents in care homes? A systematic review of qualitative and quantitative evidence. Int. J. Older People Nurs. **14**(3), e12239 (2019)
19. Leng, M., Liu, P., Zhang, P., et al.: Pet robot intervention for people with dementia: a systematic review and meta-analysis of randomized controlled trials. Psychiatry Res. **271**, 516–525 (2019)
20. Bemelmans, R., Gelderblom, G.J., Jonker, P., de Witte, L.: How to use robot interventions in intramural psychogeriatric care; A feasibility study. Appl. Nurs. Res. **30**, 154–157 (2016)
21. Jones, C., Moyle, W., Murfield, J., Draper, B., Shum, D., Beattie, E., Thalib, L.: Does cognitive impairment and agitation in dementia influence intervention effectiveness? Findings from a cluster-randomized-controlled trial with the therapeutic robot, PARO. J. Am. Med. Dir. Assoc. **19**(7), 623–626 (2018)
22. Thodberg, K., Sørensen, L.U., Videbech, P.B., Poulsen, P.H., Houbak, B., Damgaard, V., Christensen, J.W.: Behavioral responses of nursing home residents to visits from a person with a dog, a Robot Seal or aToy Cat. Anthrozoos **29**(1) (2016)
23. Portugal, D., Trindade, P., Christodoulou, E., Samaras, G., Dias, J.: On the development of a service robot for social interaction with the elderly. In: Proceedings of the IET Conference Proceedings, pp. 1–6. Institution of Engineering and Technology, London, UK (2015)

24. Melles, M., Albayrak, A., Goossens, R.: Innovating health care: key characteristics of human-centered design. International journal for quality in health care: J. Int. Soc. Qual. Health Care **33**(Supplement_1), 37–44 (2021)
25. Heerink, M., Kröse, B., Evers, V., Wielinga, B.: Assessing acceptance of assistive social agent technology by older adults: the Almere model. Int. J. Soc. Robot. **2**, 361–375 (2010)
26. Tulsulkar, G., Mishra, N., Thalmann, N.M., Lim, H.E., Lee, M.P., Cheng, S.K.: Can a humanoid social robot stimulate the interactivity of cognitively impaired elderly? A thorough study based on computer vision methods. Vis. Comput. **37**(12), 3019–3038 (2021)
27. Jøranson, N., et al.: Change in quality of life in older people with dementia participating in Paro-activity: a cluster-randomized controlled trial. J. Adv. Nurs. **72**(12), 3020–3033 (2016). https://doi.org/10.1111/jan.13076
28. Liang, A., et al.: A pilot randomized trial of a companion robot for people with dementia living in the community. J. Am. Med. Dir. Assoc. **18**(10), 871–878. (2017). https://doi.org/10.1016/j.jamda.2017.05.019
29. Jøranson, N., et al.: Effects on symptoms of agitation and depression in persons with dementia participating in robot-assisted activity: a cluster-randomized controlled trial. J. Am. Med. Dir. Assoc. **16**(10), 867–73 (2015). https://doi.org/10.1016/j.jamda.2015.05.002
30. Jones, C., et al.: Does cognitive impairment and agitation in dementia influence intervention effectiveness? Findings from a cluster-randomized-controlled trial with the therapeutic robot, PARO. J. Am. Med. Dir. Assoc. **19**(7), 623–626 (2018). https://doi.org/10.1016/j.jamda.2018.02.014
31. Moyle, W., et al.: Effect of a robotic seal on the motor activity and sleep patterns of older people with dementia, as measured by wearable technology: a cluster-randomised controlled trial. Maturitas **110**, 10–17 (2018). https://doi.org/10.1016/j.maturitas.2018.01.007
32. Kelly, P.A., et al.: The effect of PARO robotic seals for hospitalized patients with dementia: a feasibility study. Geriatr. Nurs. **42**(1), 37–45 (2021)
33. Pu, L., et al.: The effect of using PARO for people living with dementia and chronic pain: a pilot randomized controlled trial. J. Am. Med. Dir. Assoc. **21**(8), 1079–1085 (2020)
34. Moyle, W., et al.: Use of a robotic seal as a therapeutic tool to improve dementia symptoms: a cluster-randomized controlled trial. J. Am. Med. Dir. Assoc. **18**(9), 766–773 (2017). https://doi.org/10.1016/j.jamda.2017.03.018
35. Pu, L., et al.: The effect of a social robot intervention on sleep and motor activity of people living with dementia and chronic pain: a pilot randomized controlled trial. Maturitas **144**, 16–22 (2021). https://doi.org/10.1016/j.maturitas.2020.09.003
36. Chen, K., et al.: Effects of a humanoid companion robot on dementia symptoms and caregiver distress for residents in long-term care. J. Am. Med. Dir. Assoc. **21**(11), 1724–1728 (2020)
37. Park, E.-A., et al.: The humanoid robot Sil-Bot in a cognitive training program for community-dwelling elderly people with mild cognitive impairment during the COVID-19 pandemic: a randomized controlled trial. Int. J. Environ. Res. Public Health **18**(15), 8198 (3 Aug. 2021). https://doi.org/10.3390/ijerph18158198
38. Manca, M., et al.: The impact of serious games with humanoid robots on mild cognitive impairment older adults. Int. J. Hum.-Comput. Stud. **145**, 102509 (2021)
39. Whelan, S., Burke, M., Barrett, E., Mannion, A., Kovacic, T., Santorelli, A., Oliveira, B.L., Gannon, L., Shiel, E. and Casey, D.: The effects of MARIO, a social robot, on the resilience of people with dementia: a multiple case study. Gerontechnology **20** (Aug. 2020). https://doi.org/10.4017/gt.2020.20.413.10
40. Marti, P., Pollini, A., Rullo, A., Shibata, T.: Engaging with artificial pets. In: Proceedings of the Annual Conference of the European Association of Cognitive Ergonomics, September 28–October 1 2005, Creta, Greece (2005)
41. Marti, P., Palma, V., Pollini, A., Rullo, A., Shibata, T.: My gym robot. In: Proceedings of AISB 05 International Symposium on Robot Companions: Hard Problems and Open Challenges in Human-Robot Interaction, April 2005, Hatfield, UK (2005)

# Human-Centered Design to Enhance the Holter Monitor Experience for Elderly People

**Filippo Petrocchi**

## 1 Introduction

The current world is mainly characterized by an unstable context called VUCA, an acronym that stands for Volatility, Uncertainty, Complexity, and Ambiguity; the global aging phenomena and the liquid society are vastly influenced by Internet technology which is progressively more and more present in human's daily routines.

### *1.1 VUCA*

Used for the first time in 1987 in US Army War College (Pennsylvania) as an adjective to describe the volatile, uncertain, complex, and ambiguous situation generated by the end of the cold war, the term has recently been adopted in economics. In 2014, the Harvard Business Review started to recognize how the VUCA term applies in business environment too [1]. This is proven by what is happening in the current society more and more characterized by sudden changes (volatility), future unpredictability (uncertainty), situations often characterized by variables which are difficult to be analyzed (complexity) and by casual and not comprehensible relations between events (ambiguity). All these factors contribute to generate a highly unstable environment that is difficult to control by markets and industries in every sector [2, 3].

F. Petrocchi (✉)
University of Ferrara, Ferrara, Italy
e-mail: ptrfpp@unife.it

 
S. Scataglini et al. (eds.), *mHealth and Human-Centered Design Towards Enhanced Health, Care, and Well-Being*, Studies in Big Data 120,
https://doi.org/10.1007/978-981-99-3989-3_10

### 1.2 Aging Society

According to several studies, the global population will continue to grow until the end of the century, passing from almost 8 billion people today to 10.9 billion population in 2100 [4]. Furthermore, while elderly people will continue to increase the growth rate will decrease passing from the current 1,08% to the forecasted 0,1% in 2100. Those factors which are contributing to the rise of the elderly society are mainly related to the aging of the baby boomer generation (those born between 1946 and 1964) along with the increasing longevity of human beings and the decreasing birth rate [5].

In particular in Europe, according to WHO the number of people aged 65 and over is forecasted to almost double between 2010 and 2050, and the number of people aged 85 years and older is projected to rise from 14 to 19 million by 2020 and to 40 million by 2050 [6]. Last but not least the world composition will also change with a progressive decrease of young and working-aged people and a progressive increase in elderly from around 10% to around 20% [7].

### 1.3 Digitalism

Considering contemporary times, together with the VUCA conditions and the aging society, another significant factor is Digitalism.

The current world is every day increasingly turning into what can be defined as a digital world. According to ITU Statistics, (2022) 4.1 billion humans were connected to the internet in 2019 [8]. In addition, the same humans, stimulated by the crisis to provide solutions to unseen situations, had to radically change their habits and accept the digital transition by radically transforming the way they communicate, proceed, and adapt to new requirements [9].

The three factors here presented: Conditions VUCA, global aging, and digital transition contribute to generate a whole new scenario and have a deep and significant influence all over the world and in almost all economic sectors, and the healthcare field is for sure not an exception.

## 2 Healthcare Transitions

The Internet advent, the aging society, and the highly unstable VUCA conditions, coupled also with the COVID-19 pandemic crisis, have accelerated many transitions already taking place in the healthcare world.

The overall age increase along with both economic and pandemic crises has generated enormous pressure on hospital facilities, which had to consider innovative strategies to address the new, fast, and unexpected challenges that occurred in this last period.

Certainly, Internet technology has been widely adopted in this new liquid context enabling the transition of traditional services into smart ones [10]. Outpatient care is one of the clearest examples of this strategy. The outpatient strategy goal is to create parallel healthcare where preventive services are provided outside of traditional healthcare facilities [11]. Healthcare services that adopt this approach are for instance: clinical monitoring, management of chronic diseases patients, and the monitoring and prevention of people's fitness status.

Furthermore, another relevant healthcare transition is on the systemic level: from a fee-for-service system (FFS) to a Value-based System (VBS). This means a transition from an FFS system characterized by limited financial risk, limited information sharing, and limited results analysis to a VBS where information sharing, data collection, and standard protocols improve the system and provide efficient and cost-effective treatments [12].

Considering these important factors that influenced the healthcare care system, this contribution proceeds to investigate the most diffused disease categories: cardiovascular disease (CVDs).

## 3 CVDs and the HCD's Role to Innovate the Holter Monitor Experience

Cardiovascular diseases (CVDs) are globally known as a group of disorders that involves the heart and blood vessels. According to the WHO, CVDs are the most significant disease in the world since they represent 32% of all the global deaths with an estimated amount of 17.9 million people dying from that sickness [13].

In line with WHO and many national countries' policies to reduce the number of people dying from CVDs, several companies are producing and manufacturing devices to monitor and control the patient's heartbeat. Nevertheless, standard ECG devices are usually produced to accomplish budgets and economic resources and they marginally consider the user's desirability as well as the healthcare system transitions.

Human-Centered Design (HCD) is a discipline that has proven to be effective in realizing products, services, and systems that can integrate users' needs with the feasibility and viability requirements of the companies [14].

In particular, HCD is quite effective in situations with frail people like elderly people where, as Donald Norman suggests, devices are usually poorly designed since they aim to solve only functional aspects. The role of HCD is not to make devices aging-friendly but to realize artifacts that can be used also by other categories of society [15]. In this perspective, HCD contributes both to innovative products and to make the market offer more inclusive and less stigmatizing for frail groups such as elderly people.

# 4 Research Project: How to Improve Holter Monitor Experience by Human-Centered Design

In this section, the research project is presented with the illustration of the research structure and the description of each phase. The entire project follows an HCD approach, and it aims to underline the results achieved considering the specific case of the Holter monitor. To achieve this goal, a program has been set up and a research question has been formulated:

*How HCD methodologies can offer a margin for potential innovation to enhance the viability, feasibility, and desirability of the Holter monitor product experience?*

## *4.1 Methodology*

The structure of the project is characterized by a Human-Centered Design methodology where the user's needs behavior and mental models are at the core of the process at any stage together with feasibility and viability criteria.

The project was organized into 4 phases: analysis, synthesis, testing, and finalization.

As shown in Fig. 1, each step is characterized by a rhombus split into two halves: the first part, with warm colors, represents the explorative-divergent phase, and the second one, with cold colors, which illustrates the convergent phase. At the end of each phase, represented with the dashed line, it is shown the results/goal of each section. As it is possible to see in Fig. 1 after the analysis phase the result is the creation of the vision, after the synthesis phase it was produced the first version of the concept (concept v1) and after the testing phase the tested concept (concept tested v2).

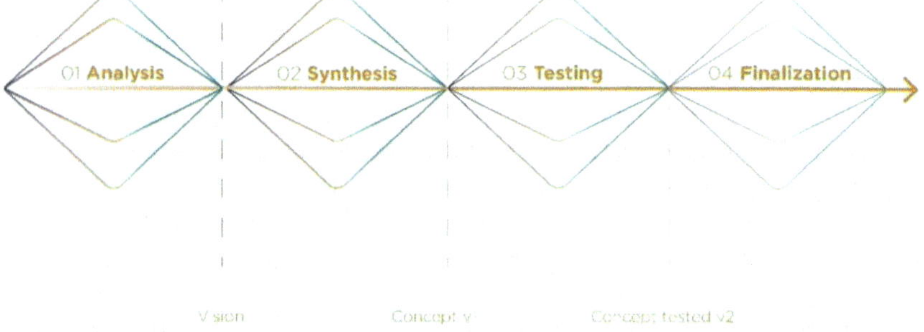


**Fig. 1** Structure of the research project

## 4.2 Phase 01—Analysis

The first part of the research project was focused on the exploration of the healthcare world with its technological transition, its business innovation, and the analysis of the user's behavior. In particular, the investigation has dived deep into the Holter monitor technology, the business related to the ECG portable devices, and the elderly needs related to the Holter monitor experience.

### 4.2.1 People

To investigate the user's perception, the starting point was the user's perspective user rather than the technological and business point of view. Considering this process, it was possible to collect a theoretical overview of the Holter monitor process with the digital materials, and then compare it with the real 24 h experience of the Holter monitor. Furthermore, to have a more complete overview of how the system around the Holter monitor was structured user and stakeholders were interviewed and their feedback was integrated into the project insights. Specifically, the following were interviewed: 14 elderly patients, 2 nurses, 1 General practitioner, and 1 Cardiologist. All the data collected in this exploration were synthesized into a visual representation as shown in Fig. 2.

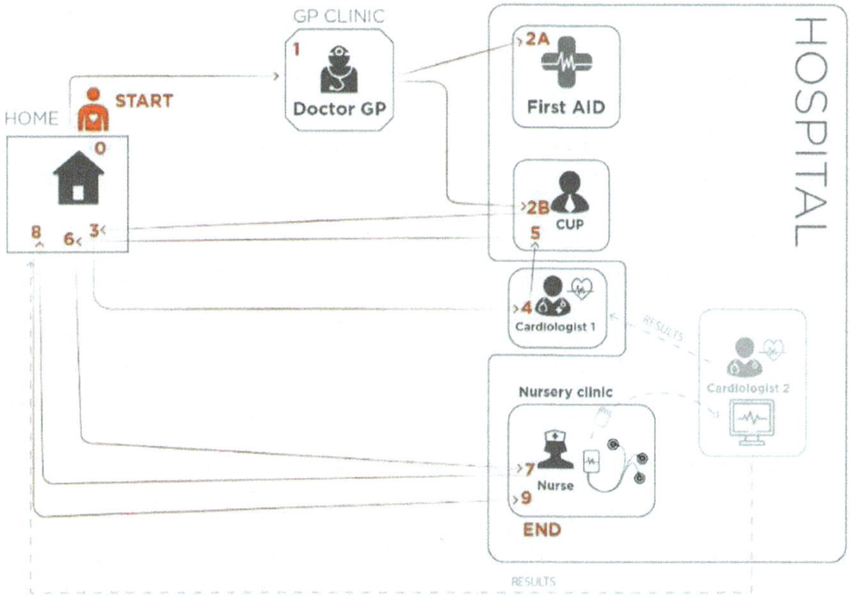


**Fig. 2** Visual representation of the system layout

From the analysis of the people section, the most important extracted insights were related to the elderly perspective, the current technology, and the overall structure of the service.

Regarding the elderly perspective, one of the most significant problems revealed during the research was related to the smartphone usability. More specifically, the mechanical and electro-mechanical generation (those born between the '40s and '60s) needed a strong effort to understand the new digital terminology usually expressed with the English language. Comparing the insights from the user's interview together with the results from the technological trends it was possible to forecast two possible future scenarios: A closer and easy-to-implement scenario where caregivers can teach elderly how to use the most recent technology. The second scenario assumes that in the future technology will be every year more and more user-friendly. Considering a time range of 5–10 years, it is fair to consider a situation where the elderly can be independent through unobtrusive and easy-to-understand technology.

Considering the Holter monitor experience, the main problems are mainly related to uncomfortable limitations such as the inability to have a shower and the skin irritation caused by the electrode's patches attached to the chest. The research also highlighted several margins of improvement by taking advantage of the digital transition which can bring many benefits in terms of efficiency. In fact, by creating online consultations it is possible to save unnecessary travel from and to the healthcare facilities. For instance, physicians can provide medical diagnoses and instructions through video calls reducing cost, cueing time, and the overall workload of the healthcare facilities.

### 4.2.2 Business

The viability of the project was also investigated. In fact, merging the trends analysis with the company profile and the research question it was possible to highlight the business scenario behind the Holter monitor device.

To begin with, it analyzed the economic size of the healthcare sector aiming to understand the level of innovation required and the related sector's leader.

Catalyzed by the pandemic crisis, the Healthcare sector has become more and more significant in those last years, and it will be central to the economic recovery with a forecasted rise prediction of 4.1% in the global healthcare spending [16]. Together with hospital facilities and government institutions, several companies are pivoting their business to make more profit, for instance, Philips or Apple. Philips after 123 years of manufacturing, sales, and development of light bulbs, in 2014 has decided to break its tradition and divide its company into healthcare and lighting. This was done to maintain the historical sector but to invest more into the more profitable healthcare field [17]. Apple as the historical manufacturer of laptops, and more recently iPad, iPhone producer has decided to invest in healthcare with apps and devices, like for instance the smartwatch, that can measure and track your level of health [18].

Narrowing down the focus from leading company to the small size company involved in the project, several interviews were taken with managers and stakeholders. Aiming to understand what was feasible in terms of business development all the innovations carried out by the research company in the last 3–5 years were analyzed. The approach of the company was more related to incremental innovation rather than radical ones. In particular, the company was at the beginning of internet technology implementation with several ECG devices and web-based applications.

An interesting insight from the business analysis was to leverage on internet and digitalism to propose a radical innovation within the company offers. In particular, the internet introduction was a clear opportunity to innovate the company's current devices by designing a less obtrusive and more efficient experience as well as a better data collection. The benefits of implementation would have been not only for the users but also for the hospital staff which could collect data in a faster, more efficient, and more organized manner.

### 4.2.3 Technology

The technological part was also investigated to complete the analysis of the Holter monitor context. First of all, the Holter monitor history and its evolution over the years were studied to understand the variable and invariable elements of the Holter monitor technology. Then the traditional models were compared with the current ECG devices available in the market.

#### Holter Monitor Evolution and Mobile Health

Since the first prototype was realized by Norman Jeffries Holter in 1947, the Holter monitor device has undergone many transformations. Observing the original device the clearest difference with the current model is the dimension and the weight: the original Holter monitor device reached the dimension of the backpack and its weight was 38 kg.

Over the years, technology development has enabled dimension reduction as well as the improvement and the safety of the data collected. Nevertheless, besides the technological development of the device, the current Holter monitor still presents several challenges with cables, electrodes, data collection, and data analysis as well as psychological and physical comfort issues [19–21].

A promising solution that can address most of these issues is the biosensors which have the potential, in the future, to replace traditional Holter monitors. The success of the biosensors is mainly due to their small size appearance with better or the same level of signal acquisition compared to a standard Holter monitor [22].

The rise of the biosensor can be also linked with a more systemic technological transition: the shift toward mobile health.

As shown in Fig. 3, the mobile health applied to the Heart prevention is characterized by a wearable ECG device that continuously transmits data to the mobile

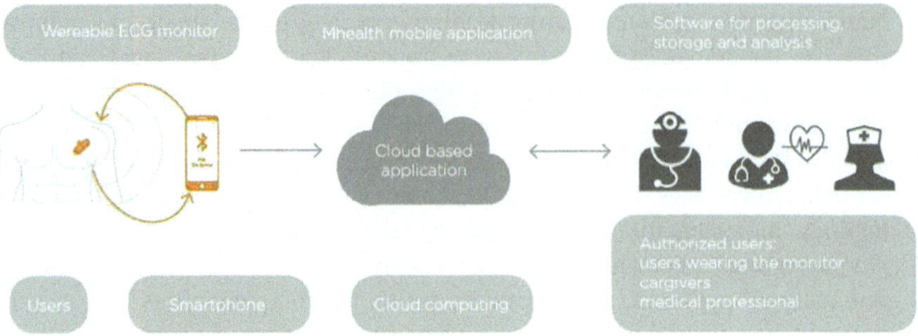


**Fig. 3** Visual representation of the mobile health

application which constantly safely transmits data to the cloud. All the data are then stored in the cloud which is accessible only to a specific group of people such as caregivers, physicians, or the patient themselves [19].

The rise of the mobile health can be explained by several reasons such as the strong demand of the healthcare system for cheaper and more effective healthcare, the intention for a higher quality of life, the increasing patient mobility, the health awareness as well as the involvement of ICT (information communication technology). Furthermore, the ICT involvement in the healthcare system presents the high potential to enable remote monitoring, remote monitoring, remote care, and other healthcare remote services which can reduce the pressure on healthcare facilities.

In addition, mobile health represents the opportunity to tailor the healthcare services to customers' needs and to optimize unnecessary operations such as data collection. Nevertheless, this new configuration necessitates working together with a strong cyber security system since the data collected contain sensitive contents that should be accessible only to the users and their physicians.

## Commercial ECG System

Together with the chronological evolution of the Holter monitor and the rise of mobile health, it investigated the current panorama of Commercial ECG solutions. The scope of the investigation was to extract innovation opportunities to implement them in the future Holter monitor device. A structure of five different categories was adopted to organize the vast number of devices present in the current ECG market. The five categories selected were patch solution, handheld solution, Holter monitor case, wearable body contact, and invasive devices.

The analysis involved more than 50 solutions, and it was useful to individuate the key feature of the Holter monitor experience as well as the common pitfalls and weaknesses. Some of the most important key features highlighted were the shape and dimension of sensors and devices; the IoT integration, the waterproof features, and the possibility to set up the device by the user itself. The key weaknesses were the limited battery duration, the difficulty to keep the device attached to the body, the irritation caused by the patches, and the interface understanding difficulties.

An interesting result of this analysis was the ability to understand which device was more innovative and closer to mobile health and which was less innovative and more connected to traditional healthcare.

### 4.2.4 Conclusion of the Research

By completing the analysis of the three pillars of industrial design (Usability, Viability, Feasibility) it was possible to formulate a new business strategy, an innovative system layout, and a technology implementation plan.

#### A New Business Strategy

Comparing the different solutions available in the market with the product selected by the company as a starting point, it was clear that the product itself needed a new design cheaper and less obtrusive. As shown in Fig. 4, the new strategy consists of moving from a quite obtrusive and expensive product to a more comfortable and affordable one.

#### An Innovative System Layout

The analysis of the system layout summarized in the previous chapter in Fig. 2 had highlighted many unnecessary steps in the Holter monitor experience. Merging the promising trends of mobile health with the opportunity of re-design the Holter monitor experience, it was created a completely new system characterized by the creation of two strictly linked circles: the circle of family made of caregivers and parents and the circle of experts mainly characterized by professionals such as physicians and nurses.

In this system, see Fig. 5, data are collected utilizing the smartphone, and data are stored in the cloud which is accessible only by specific medical professionals and by the user.

#### Technology Implementation Plan

A technology implementation plan was elaborated merging the current product with the most promising current trends and elaborating 4 levels of implementation. The first level consisted in reducing dimensions by miniaturized elements and removing large elements such as the LCD. The second level of implementation was a wireless device characterized by patches, electrodes, and the data cloud designed as main

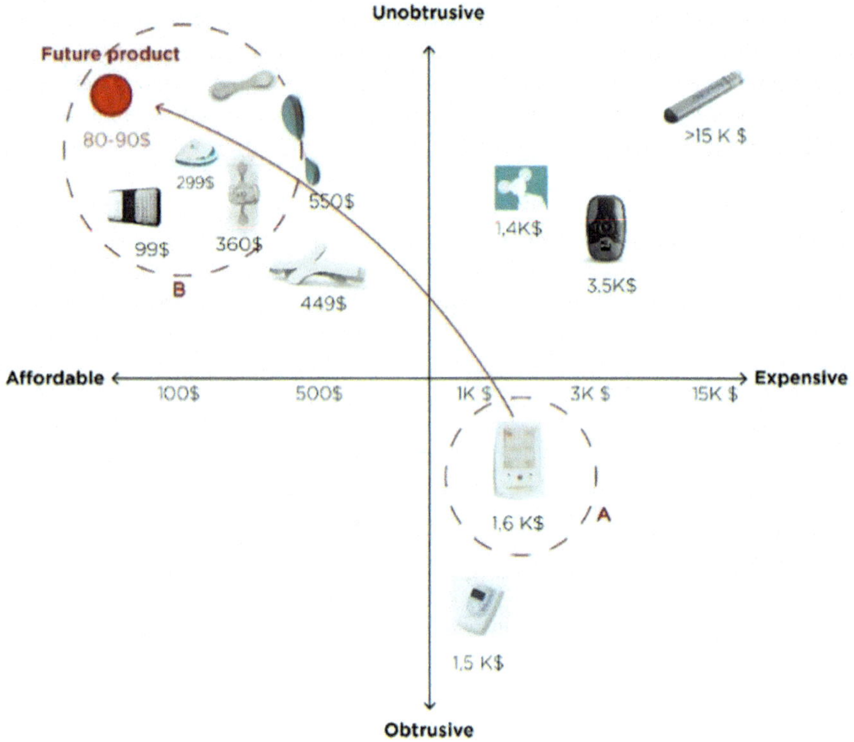


Fig. 4 Visual representation of the new business strategy

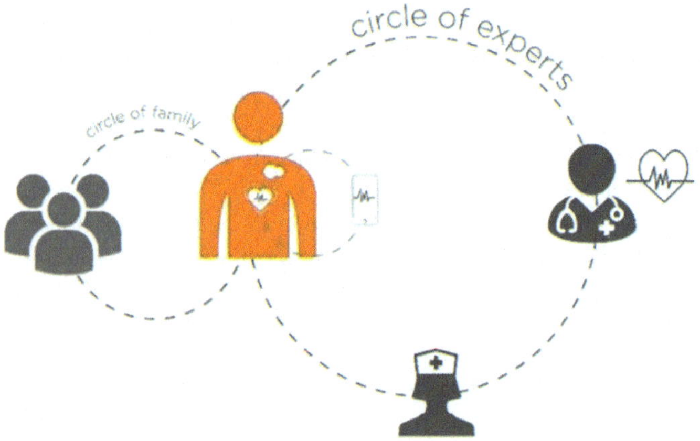


Fig. 5 The new system layout

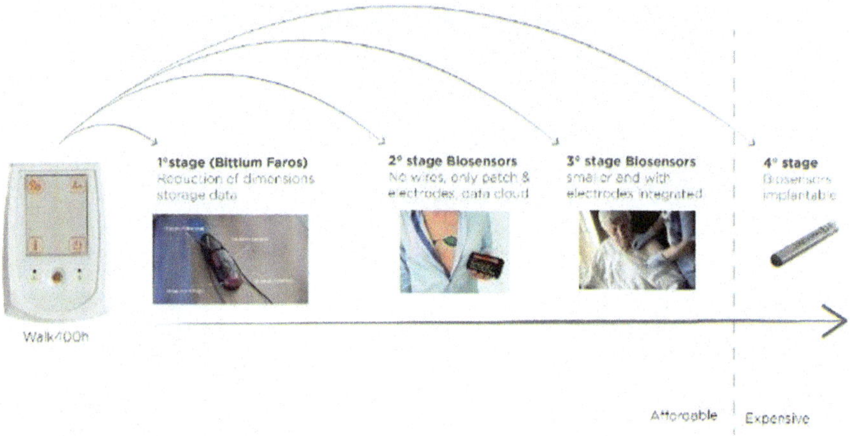


**Fig. 6** The four levels of technology implementation plan

data storage. The third stage went a level further by the integration of all the components in a flexible solution. Finally, a more radical scenario was considered with an implantable solution (see Fig. 6).

## 4.3 *Synthesis*

Once completed the research part, the goal of the next phase was to transform the research insights into a product-service concept. Firstly, a list of requirements was elaborated, then a brainstorming session about the most important issues was organized. All the data collected from the list of requirements and the brainstorming session were then collected and elaborated into three concepts. Those three concepts were presented and discussed and critically evaluated with the Harris profile matrix and the stakeholder feedback. To conclude the concept phase, a final result was elaborated further merging several aspects of the three concept presented and finalizing some additional features.

### 4.3.1 List of Requirements

The first step of the synthesis phase was to create the list of requirements to focus on all the features needed by the new device, specifying which were the "hard" primary requirements and which were the "soft" secondary requirements. Together with the list of requirements, also evaluation criteria were defined.

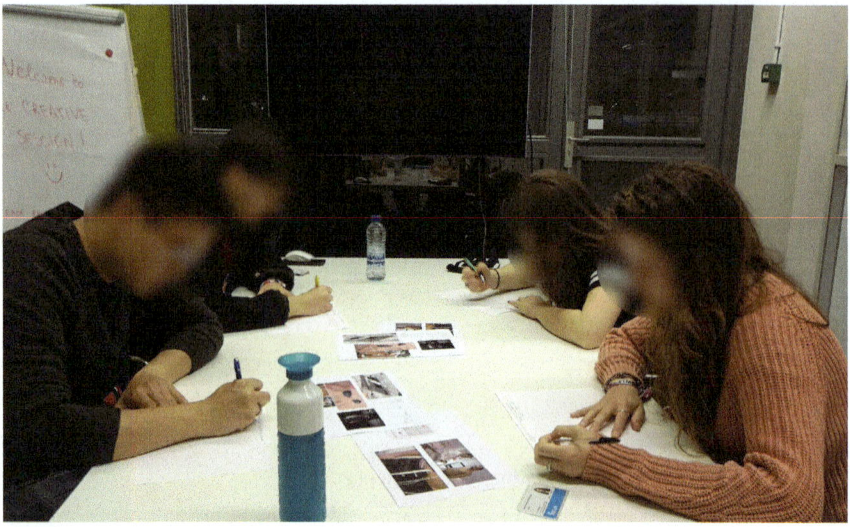

**Fig. 7** Brainstorming session about critical situations of the holter monitor experience

### 4.3.2 Brainstorming Session

Aiming to combine rational with intuitive thinking, a brainstorming session was organized immediately after the list of requirements. Considering the critical points of the Holter monitor experience, during the brainstorming session it was asked four people with four different backgrounds to solve four main critical situations.

The brainstorming session was organized in 10-min turns where the participants tried to solve the proposed issues by sketching or written text. Stimuli were provided in the form of photography, and at the end of each session, results were discussed, confronted, and collected. Among the many touch points of the Holter monitor experience, the investigated aspects during the brainstorming were: how to inform the patient about the procedure; how to check the correct functioning of the Holter monitor; how to communicate eventual problems during the process; how to avoid skin irritation; how to use the device while having a shower (see Fig. 7).

### 4.3.3 Concept Proposal

Combining the list of requirements with the brainstorming results three concepts were elaborated and presented as shown in Fig. 8. During the session priority was given to originality and future perspectives to collect the most innovative ideas with the widest variety.

Three-concept were proposed with a special focus on their unique selling point (USP) and their benefits for the user.

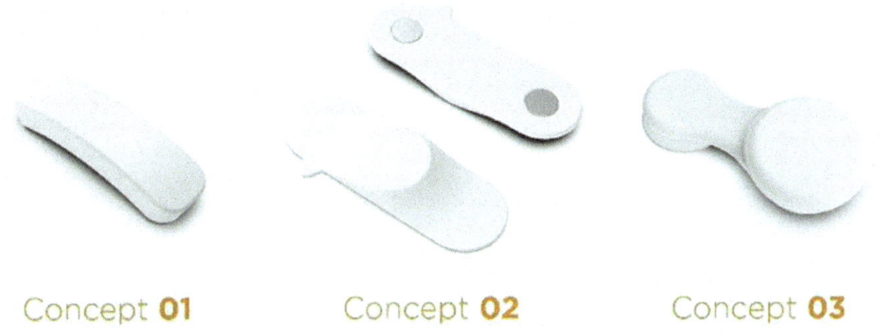


**Fig. 8** The three concepts

Concept 01, the Holter belt monitor concept could collect the user's heartbeat using dry electrodes which periodically transmit data to the cloud through the smartphone. The USP of this concept was the total absence of patches which solved itching and skin irritation issues.

The Flexible patch concept, concept two in Fig. 8, was a flexible wireless ECG device able to measure and to transmit the user's heartbeat to the cloud by using a smartphone as a gateway. As the name suggests, its peculiarity is to be flexible and adaptable to the user's body resulting in a more comfortable and less obtrusive device.

The last concept, concept three, is a Holter case concept attached to the body with standard electrode patches. The concept could be considered the most feasible since it was very close to the production manner of the company involved in the research project.

### 4.3.4 Concept Evaluation

Once the elaboration of the three concepts was complete the divergence phase ended, and it started the convergence phase. To narrow the three concepts to one and select the most promising solution it was used the Harris profile matrix, as shown in Fig. 9.

Considering the criteria selected at the beginning of the synthesis phase each criterion was given a score with + (if the concept meets the criteria), ++ if brilliantly meets the criteria, and − if badly meets the criteria. In the end, the concept that resulted as more promising was the flexible patch far followed by the Holter case concept and the Holter belt concept.

### 4.3.5 Final Concept V1

To achieve the final concept of the synthesis phase, several iterations were conducted aiming to merging the flexible patch concept with the Holter case. Furthermore,

| | Concept01 | Concept02 | Concept03 |
|---|---|---|---|
| Comfort | ++ | + | ++ |
| Dimension | + | + | + |
| Flexibility | ++ | - | + |
| Reliability | + | - | + |
| Cost | + | - | ++ |
| Manegeability | + | - | + |
| Waterproof | + | ++ | - |
| Cleanability | + | ++ | - |
| Environment | - | ++ | - |
| Setting up | ++ | - | + |
| | | | |
| Final Score | 12+ 1- | 8+ 5- | 9+ 3- |

**Fig. 9** Harris profile matrix

special attention was given to the user experience and to the setting up phase designed to make older people as independent as possible while installing the device.

## *4.4 Testing*

To verify the validity of the previously discussed concept, a usability test was organized. Among all the possible aspects of the HM, it was decided to focus on the setting up phase since during this aspect the most relevant interactions occurred between the device and the user.

### 4.4.1 Usability Test

The test focus was both to determine the device's usability and to understand what kind of problems could arise while approaching the setting phase. In particular, the research question of the usability test was

*Which aspect of the product and which one of the users influence the setting up phase?*

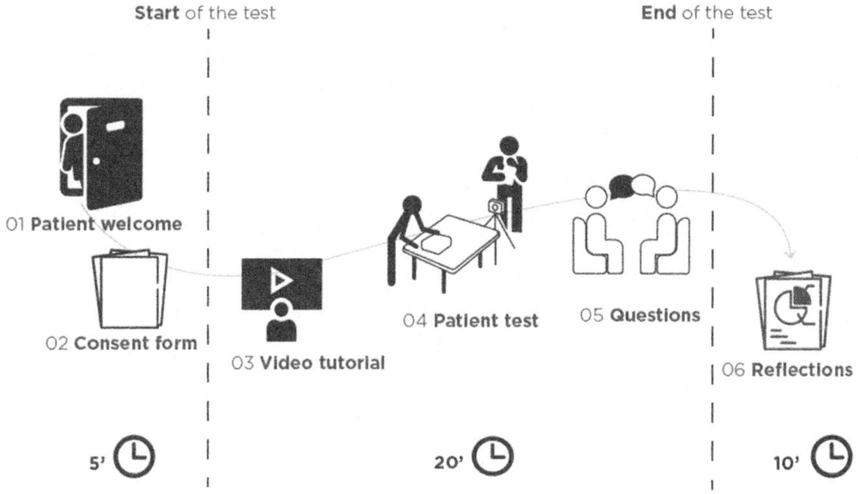


**Fig. 10** Schematic representation of the test

### 4.4.2 Test Structure

Before the actual test, a pilot test was set up and performed that everything was manageable in the prearranged time. The pilot test confirmed what was planned a head with a few little variations in the structure of the test. As shown in Fig. 10, the final test was structured in three parts. The welcoming part, the actual test, and the final part with reflections.

In the first part, patients were first welcomed and then instructed on how to fill out the consent form. In the same section, a video tutorial was shown to illustrate all the steps necessary to complete the user test. Once patients viewed the video, the real test was performed by completing tasks, and notes were taken by an observer with special attention when hesitations occurred. Then specific questions were asked about the device. The last part was then characterized by user's reflections on the overall experience with a special attention on matching and mismatching interactions during the test.

### 4.4.3 Test Results and Concept Improvements

Overall, the test was performed by 5 people aged between 65 and 80 years old. All the tests were completed both in a hospital and in a domestic environment. Through this usability test, it was possible to acquire many insights into the user's perception, the device and docking station usability, and the instruction given with the prototyped application.

Regarding users, a significant difference was noticed between people aged 65 and those aged 80. The former group was quite familiar with the technology while people in their 80s were having difficulties not only with smartphones but also with technological terms usually expressed in the English language. However, by providing some help and translating the technical terms into their language both groups were able to complete all the procedure.

As far as the device and the instructions, patients preferred to hold the device in their hands rather than use the designated seat. The main reason was related to the instability of the prototype which was missing grip with the table, and it usually slipped away from its housing.

Concerning the app, the main result was that patient performance instructions were already acquired from the video and they use the different steps in the app as a checker or they did not use it at all. Furthermore, the test also revealed some hesitation moments in several app screens. Those hesitations were used afterwards to enhance the concept and to improve the match between user expectations and user goals.

## 5 Results

Implementing all the suggestions and feedback from the user test into the concept elaborated, it was possible to define the final concept. A Holter monitor product system was perceived as more comfortable and less obtrusive for elderly people, more competitive on the related market, in line with the company profile, and feasible to the point of realizing a pre-production prototype (see Fig. 11).

A more detailed overview of the final results is provided in Fig. 12 where a visual representation was made to make more understandable the level of definition achieved.

As far as concerns the device desirability, the new concept could be considered more competitive from the reference starting point since a 70% reduction in terms of volume and weight was achieved. Translating these technical features in user's terms, the reduced weight and dimension of the device make the new concept way more comfortable than the starting device consequently increasing the user's acceptance time. In addition, the comfort was increased also by the wire's removal and by the longer battery autonomy. Such features enabled the user to create the newly designed system removing all the unnecessary trips from and to the hospital normally used to complete tasks such as the setup, data unload, or battery charging. Furthermore, the lack of wires provided the user more freedom to move further extending the acceptance period and the overall comfort. Regarding the viability, the concept is in line with the strategic vision of the company and at the same time it opens up future strategic scenarios. As far as what concerns feasibility, the new concept was developed to the point of a pre-production prototype. This means that the prototype reached the level of definition of the last step before the production. Reaching this level, it was possible to test the ability to record the human ECG and transmit it to the smartphone by means of Bluetooth technology.

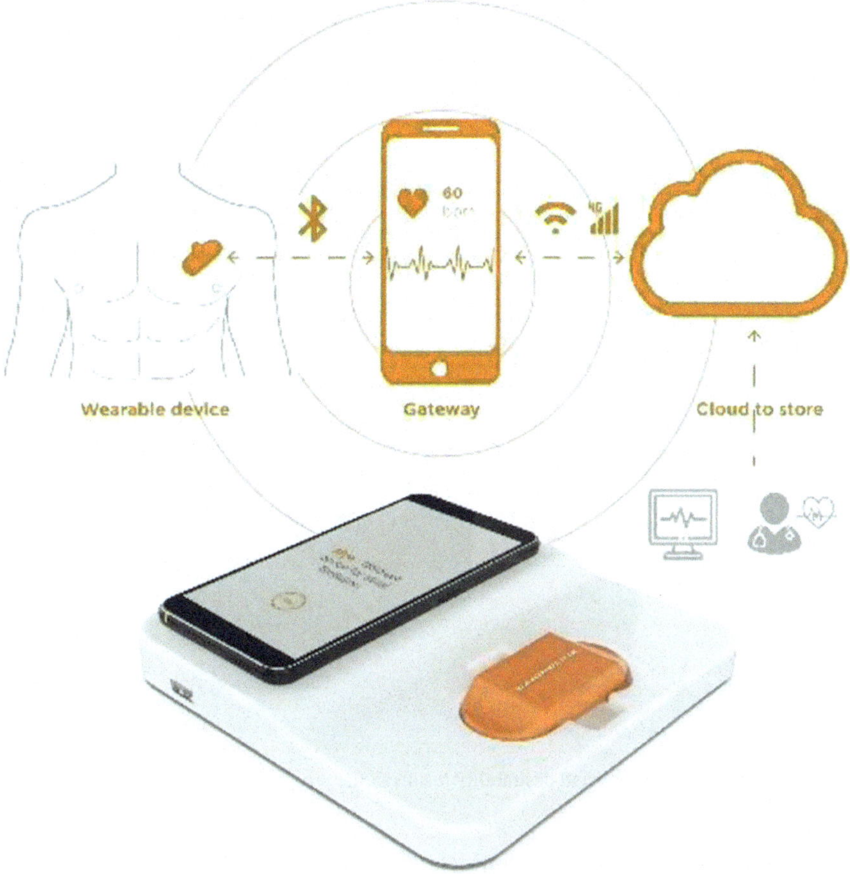


**Fig. 11** Representation of the final outputs project: Final system layout, docking station, app, and device

## 6 Conclusion

Considering the whole project, it is possible to affirm that Human Centered Design (HCD) is a contemporary approach able to solve current and significant issues in a healthcare context, and more specifically within the frame of the Holter monitor experience.

Project results have proven the Human-Centered Methodology's effectiveness to face healthcare challenges by implementing the user's feedback at any stage of the project. Furthermore, the approach achieved potential improvements not only in terms of desirability but also on the side of viability and feasibility.

The main reason for this success can be related to the fit of the HCD method with the current context of VUCA conditions, Digitalization, and Aging society.

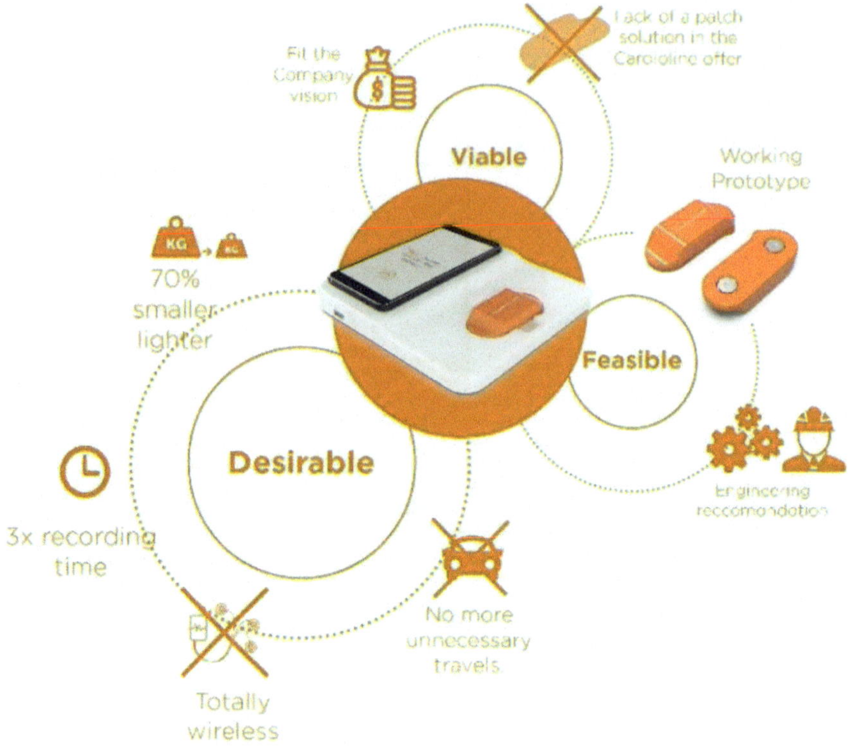


**Fig. 12** Viability, feasibility, and desirability results of the project

To solve VUCA conditions, which means unstable, volatile complex, and ambiguous situations a new and innovative methodology is needed. HCD can be taken into account since it is flexible and open to user's feedback.

Regarding the aging society, HCD can be considered a promising tool to face challenges related to the rising of the aging society. This is mainly because HCD is a discipline based on the analysis of behavior, mental models, and the context of the user.

Concerning Digitalization, the current affirmation of ICT and internet technology are pushing the boundary of product customization by tailoring the service on the behavior, mental models, and user needs. HCD seems very useful to extract user's needs, feedback, and opinions and implementing those insights from the user at any stage of the project.

Finally, it is also important to highlight several insights regarding elderly people. Aged people are an important category to study since not only they are expected to grow in the future, but also because the entire society can benefit from a more aware knowledge of their wellness. In addition, the category of elderly is interesting and difficult to analyze since they are not all the same. Being the same age is very significant only when it comes to the probability to have some health issues, but their mental models and behaviors change person by person.

Considering this vision, the contribution aims to challenge the mainstream definition of an elderly person considered as a slower people who need more time to process and actuate tasks. In fact, with this research, it was possible to define elderly as people who need different interactions between their mind and routines, and between their physical needs and product, service, and systems. A different interaction is of remarkable importance since elderly are also less prone to errors and alternative scenarios.

To conclude, the current scenario while approached with the correct methodology can be considered a promising situation to create inclusive environments also for elderly people. A scenario where more and more automation is becoming a tool to help frail people like elderly to maintain and sustain their independence.

## References


1. Turi, D.: What Is VUCA and Why Innovating Is Even More Important Today? (2022). https://studiozao.com/resources/what-is-vuca-and-why-innovating-is-important-today. Accessed 30 May 2022
2. Kraaijenbrink, J.: What Does VUCA Really Mean? (2018). https://www.forbes.com/sites/jeroenkraaijenbrink/2018/12/19/what-does-vuca-really-mean/?sh=6a5f465417d6. Accessed 31 Jan. 2021
3. Bennett, N., Lemoine, G.: What VUCA Means for You (2014). https://hbr.org/2014/01/what-vuca-really-means-for-you. Accessed 11 Feb. 2021
4. Roser, M.: Future population growth. Our world in data (2013)
5. Fatima, K., Moridpour, S.: Measuring public transport accessibility for the elderly. In: MATEC Web of Conferences, vol. 259, p. 03006. EDP Sciences (2019)
6. WHO Healthy Ageing Data and Statistics (2020). https://www.euro.who.int/en/health-topics/Life-stages/healthy-ageing/data-and-statistics
7. Hannah Ritchie and Max Roser: Age Structure. Published online at OurWorldInData.org. (2019). https://ourworldindata.org/age-structure
8. ITU Statistics: (2022). https://www.itu.int/en/ITU-D/Statistics/Pages/stat/default.aspx. Accessed 30 May 2022
9. ITU: Ageing in a digital world–from vulnerable to valuable, pp. 10–11 (2021). https://epale.ec.europa.eu/system/files/2021-07/Ageing%20in%20a%20digital%20world%20%20from%20vulnerable%20to%20valuable.pdf
10. Active Advice: What is Smart Health and How do People Benefit? (2017). https://www.activeadvice.eu/news/concept-projects/what-is-smart-healthand-how-do-people-benefit/
11. Digital Deloitte: Survey of US health system CEOs: Moving forward in an uncertain environment (2017). https://www2.deloitte.com/content/dam/Deloitte/us/Documents/life-sciences-health-care/us-lshc-ch3-margin-pressure-and-the-search-for-new-revenue-streams.pdf
12. Digital Deloitte: 2018 Global health care outlook (2018). https://www2.deloitte.com/content/dam/Deloitte/tw/Documents/life-sciences-healthcare/tw-lshc-hc-outlook-2018.pdf
13. WHO: Cardiovascular diseases (CVDs) (2022). https://www.who.int/news-room/fact-sheets/detail/cardiovascular-diseases-(cvds). Accessed 2 June 2022
14. Petrocchi, F.: How to enhance elderly care products, services, and systems by means of IoT technology and human-centered design approach. In: Internet of Things for Human-Centered Design, pp. 63–72. Springer, Singapore (2022)

15. NN Group: Design for elderly [Video] (2021). https://www.youtube.com/watch?v=uP6IbeggAeo
16. Economist Intelligence Unit: Healthcare in 2022 (2021)
17. Mocker, M., Ross, J.: Transforming Royal Philips to reinvent healthcare in the digital age: case study (2017)
18. CBInsights: Apple is going after the health care industry, starting with personal health data (2019). https://www.cbinsights.com/research/apple-healthcare-strategy-apps/
19. Trobec, R., et al.: Body Sensors and Electrocardiography (2018)
20. Lee, S.P., Ha, G., Wright, D.E., Ma, Y., Sen-Gupta, E., Haubrich, N.R., et al.: Highly flexible, wearable, and disposable cardiac biosensors for remote and ambulatory monitoring. npj Digit. Med. **1**(1), 2 (2018)
21. Frakt, A.: What i learned while i wear a heart monitor. The New York Times (2018). https://www.nytimes.com/2015/09/15/upshot/what-i-learnedwhile-wearing-a-heart-monitor.html
22. Barrett, P.M., Komatireddy, R., Haaser, S., Topol, S., Sheard, J., Encinas, J., Topol, E.J.: Comparison of 24-hour Holter monitoring with 14-day novel adhesive patch electrocardiographic monitoring. Am. J. Med.**127**(1), 95-e11 (2014)

# Exploring a Configurable Virtual Environment for the Assessment and Diagnosis of the Driver's Psychophysical State

**Jessica Longhin, Andrea Amidei, and Gian Andrea Giacobone**

## 1 Introduction[1]

One of the leading causes of death around the world is road accidents. As reported by the World Health Organization (WHO) in one of its latest reports [1], this fact occupies the 8th place for the highest number of deaths each year. The causes are mainly linked to human driving errors [2] that can be affected by many different causal factors, such as driving personal issues, inadequate knowledge, training or skills, impairments, willful behaviors, infrastructure, and environmental problems [3]. Among these, the most significant elements are related to the human physiological and psychological conditions and states because a considerable part of road accidents is caused by stress, inattention, and fatigue when driving. That is because

[1] The contribution was conceived, written and reviewed jointly by the authors. Gian Andrea Giacobone produced the entire section "*1 Introduction*". Andrea Amidei is responsible for subsections "*3.3 The design of a system to collect and analyze users' biometric data*" and "*4.2 KSS and biometric values*". Jessica Longhin is responsible for the entire sections "*2 Virtual Environment*", "*3 Methodology and Approach*", and "*4 Results*", excluding the subparts written by Andrea. Section "*4.4 Future works*" was jointly written by Jessica and Andrea. Lastly, the "*5 Conclusions*" section was jointly written by the three authors.

J. Longhin · G. A. Giacobone (✉)
Department of Architecture, University of Ferrara, Via Quartieri, 8, 44121 Ferrara, Italy
e-mail: gianandrea.giacobone@unife.it

J. Longhin
e-mail: jessica.longhin@edu.unife.it

A. Amidei
Department of Engineering "Enzo Ferrari", University of Modena and Reggio Emilia, Via P. Vivarelli, 10, 41125 Modena, Italy
e-mail: andrea.amidei@unimore.it



S. Scataglini et al. (eds.), *mHealth and Human-Centered Design Towards Enhanced Health, Care, and Well-Being*, Studies in Big Data 120,
https://doi.org/10.1007/978-981-99-3989-3_11

the phenomenon of road accidents comes from the intersection of two main factors related to the cognitive capabilities and limitations of the human brain.

The first aspect is that the act of driving is inherently a highly complex skill that requires the sustained supervising of multiple and integrated perceptual and cognitive inputs [4] or monitoring the dynamic and ever-changing environment and enhancing situation awareness [5], but also for rapidly processing the various cognitive operations of perception, decision, and reaction that are necessary to react promptly to a driving event [6].

The second factor is that the cognitive capacities of humans are limited and selective, as the human brain cannot process a high amount of multiple sensory information simultaneously [7]. The limited attentional capability divides attention among all competing sensory inputs and could adversely affect the driver's performance. That is because, most of the time, those limitations can lead to road accidents.

Moreover, nowadays, attentional limitations on driver performance are aggravated by the increasing proliferation of complex in-vehicle technologies that can deteriorate the primary driving performance through additional secondary tasks, for instance, by using GPS (Global Positioning System) navigation systems [8], mobile telecommunications [9, 10], or even sophisticate sound systems [11, 12].

Besides, in terms of Human–Machine Interaction (HMI), another high source of distraction is generated by the proliferation of new advanced in-vehicle interfaces that are currently transforming the majority of driving information into visual elements [13, 14], which, in turn, require a high level of visual demands even while driving the vehicle [15]. That is because, nowadays, the high number of driving-related interactions increases the complexity of modern vehicles, which requires an increasing number of elements and controls that must be displayed on a vehicle dashboard by law [16]. Those aspects inevitably move vehicle information into interactive and touchscreen displays, which, although they can create a cleaner and less cluttered design [17], are complex to learn and use [18], and cause visual informational overload among many drivers [12, 15, 19].

Although sophisticated assistive driving technologies are progressively evolving to better assist driver control in preventing and/or recovering from human errors during dangerous situations [20, 21], cognitive attention and human management must not be overlooked. That is because the multiple competing sensory inputs continue to have a demanding weight on the limited cognitive resources of the drivers [14]. For instance, low levels of autonomous driving still require attentive drivers because, even though the vehicle can drive autonomously for the majority of the time, human control must be present to monitor the status of the vehicle's system continuously. That allows the driver to be prepared to intervene in an uncontrolled situation [22].

Considering that, it is possible to identify distracting activities—associated with driver inattention, fatigue, and drowsiness—as one of the leading causes of vehicular accidents [23]. For this reason, analyzing those human-related factors helps to better study the causes and the effects of particular physiological and psychological states on driving performance to ensure safer and better driving. In particular, this contribution focuses on predicting the effects of drowsiness, experimenting with and validating technologies that can detect and/or predict sleepiness.

## *1.1 The Drowsy Driving Problems*

Driver drowsiness is the dangerous combination of driving and sleepiness or fatigue. Generally, drowsiness can be considered the intermediate state between wakefulness and being asleep [24]. Thus, the corresponding experience determines a synonym for fighting against falling asleep.

As indicated by the past literature [25], driver drowsiness refers to a multi-dimensional concept that includes physical and mental fatigue, and sleepiness. The latter refers to people's difficulties staying awake and disappears only after sleep. Instead, physical and mental fatigue is a cumulative process of a continuous task, which can provoke cognitive impairments when performing a given activity. It fades after a period of rest. Considering that the main fatigue symptoms can be associated with difficulties in maintaining focus, vigilance, attention, concentration, or staying awake. Moreover, the higher the level of fatigue, the higher the chance of provoking microsleep, in which the driver becomes unconscious for a fraction that could come from 500 ms to 30 s [25].

Of course, both elements represent a high risk for road safety when manifesting at the wheel. Many studies consider driver drowsiness as one of the common factors causing traffic accidents [26], accounting for 20% of all severe and fatal crashes [25, 27].

Several factors can lead to driver drowsiness. Following the study of May and Baldwin [28], it is possible to categorize the causal factors that affect drowsiness into two main categories: sleep-related and task-related fatigue.

The first category refers to sleep disorders, deprivation, or restriction. Every human has a circadian rhythm, an internal and iterative biological clock. It regulates the sleep–wake alternation during the day and may include a loss of attentiveness in the early afternoon when people are sleepier [29]. Since the human's physiological rhythm is programmed to facilitate sleep onset at these moments, a high rate of those accidents occurs during the afternoon or night [30].

While sleep disorder or deprivation occurs when a body does not get enough sleep. This lack of sleep creates a sleep debt that expands over time to the point where our minds will automatically shut down. Those sleep-related factors could be influenced by biological and physiological parameters, like age, gender, health status, chronic diseases, or ingestion of substances, which can significantly affect sleep conditions and the tendency of people to become drowsier drivers [25].

The second category depends on the combination of driving tasks and the driving environment. Active factors can include high traffic density, poor visibility, or being required to perform an auxiliary secondary task in addition to driving [31, 32]. Passive factors are associated with underloading driving conditions—for instance, driving in monotonous environments for long periods or during partially or completely automated driving tasks [31]—which can be influenced by landscape monotony [26], traffic conditions [33], roadway geometry [34], light settings [35], and again, time of the journey [36].

Finally, to moderate the risk associated with drowsiness, many different measurement protocols and technologies have been developed in the past years to help researchers collect data in this field. As Soares, Ferreira, and Couto report in their study [25], driver drowsiness can be measured and assessed through many different variables associated with

- Physiological parameters, like eye and eyelid movements, degree of eye-opening, signs of longer blink duration, nodding, yawning, and a drooping posture.
- Driving performance, such as reaction time, steering entropy for measuring situated safety margins, speed, lateral lane tracking, and following headway.
- Drowsiness subjective measures based on the NASA-Task Load Index, Stanford Sleepiness Scale (SSS), Sleepiness Symptoms Questionnaire (SSQ), Borg Rating of Perceived Exertion (BORG), Karolinska Sleepiness Scale (KSS).
- Full driver tracking is based on eye tracking, facial expression or features, skin conductance, brain waves, and heart rate.

## *1.2 Challenges and Opportunities of Studying Drowsy Driving*

Collecting data on driver drowsiness is crucial in developing a prevention system to reduce and prevent road accidents related to this topic. The most realistic environment is naturally the real world, though, carrying out drowsiness measurements in that scenario would be impractical because some weather, road, or traffic conditions may be unpredictable to control. In addition, due to ethical reasons, performing some experiments in the physical world is dangerous or impossible to conduct.

A test track can provide a safer environment and the possibility of giving test drivers more equal conditions. On the contrary, it lacks realism [37].

For these reasons, a driving simulator is a good solution that can simulate perfectly the characteristics of a realistic environment, in which test conditions for measuring fatigue can be controlled and varied safely.

The driving simulator imitates the act of driving a real car. It has a set of physical features, including a driving seat, a steering wheel, pedals, vehicle controls, a sound system, and a virtual windshield with screens to display the virtual surroundings [38]. Ensuring a valid representation of real driving must guarantee realistic performance and behaviors of the generated environment [37].

For many decades, a driving simulator has been utilized to study driving behaviors and now is the most adapted tool to investigate drowsiness and its related effects on driving performance.

A driving simulator presents many advantages to these typologies of scientific research because it avoids unexpected and dangerous events. In addition, a well-controlled environment allows researchers to standardize their measurement methods because they are easy to control and reproduce [25]. That is because the software can modify the experimental conditions of a given scenario to provoke fatigue and sleepiness in drivers without putting them in hazardous driving situations. Furthermore, using a driving simulator facilitates collecting data offering a more precise measurement of driving performance [39] because the driving system can connect itself to other technological devices that can merge the physiological parameters of the driver with the environmental data of the virtual scenario.

Considering that, the contribution focuses on developing an open-source driving simulator, specifically conceived to help researchers to investigate the relation between drive drowsiness and the psychophysical state of drives through the use of a flexible and customizable virtual environment. The research objective is to create a driving simulator with a series of configurable variables and scalable parameters that allows researchers to set up the environment freely according to their research needs. The final aim is to maintain the characteristics of the real environment as similar as possible to the real world, to collect reliable data while keeping the driver in a safe and secure environment.

## 2 Virtual Environment

To start developing the driving simulator, the study investigated how to program and render a virtual environment through the use of a game engine. The latter is a specific program that enables individuals or companies to create a virtual game. It provides a series of different features and is responsible for running the graphics, checking the physics of the actions, administrating the internal memory system, and other features necessary to build a reliable environment to run the game.

The general idea behind the software of game engines is to create a common and universal framework that can be used for the creation of any type of game. This software is made of reusable components that developers can use to create the interface of the game. Each engine consists of six fundamental features, common to all software:

1. Input;
2. Graphic/Rendering Engine;
3. Physics Engine;
4. Artificial Intelligence;
5. Sound/Audio Engine;
6. Networking.

To date, many game engines are viable on the market, each of which is optimized for the use of a specific platform, be it a computer, a console, a mobile device, or a Virtual Reality Headset. For this contribution, the research study analyzed several common game engines that are utilized mostly for the development of virtual games for platforms, such as computers, PlayStation, and Xbox. The research identified Unreal Engine and Unity as the two most common game engines widely used among developers. Their main characteristics are

1. Unreal Engine is essentially a multi-platform engine for developing games that helps use real-time technology to transform ideas into visual products. Its peculiarity is the ability to be adaptable to many different games to make possible the creation of unique experiences. The game engine requires skilled developers with a great experience.
2. Unity has similar characteristics as the previous game engine, but it allows the developers to create interactive elements (both in 2D and 3D), with ease. The user interface is easy to learn, reducing time, and costs for training. It has excellent functionality, high-quality content, and the ability to be used for any typology of a virtual game. The Unity Store also provides a vast collection of plug-ins and content that facilitates developers to assemble complex environments.

From their analysis, Unity appears as the most easily accessible and easy-to-learn software, however, it is not optimized and designed to create a realistic simulation environment, in which graphics and physics must be as real and realistic as possible. Consequently, the choice must necessarily fall on Unreal Engine.

## 3 Methodology and Approach

For the application of these concepts, a theoretical case study was created through the collaboration between the University of Ferrara and the University of Modena and Reggio Emilia, Italy. The goal of this project was the creation of a driving simulator for the collection of data relating to drowsiness and the subsequent analysis of these to extrapolate useful data for prevention (see Fig. 1).

This work process followed three main research activities:

1. The design, creation, and programming of the driving simulator;
2. The programming of the application for the collection of data concerning drowsiness;
3. The design of a system to collect and analyze users' biometric data.

### *3.1 The Design, Creation, and Programming of the Driving Simulator*

As for the first step, the design started with the analysis of the existing virtual environments. The aim was to highlight the strengths and gaps of what is already on the market to extrapolate the requirements that our simulator should have met.

**Fig. 1** Block system for the synthesis of methodological procedures

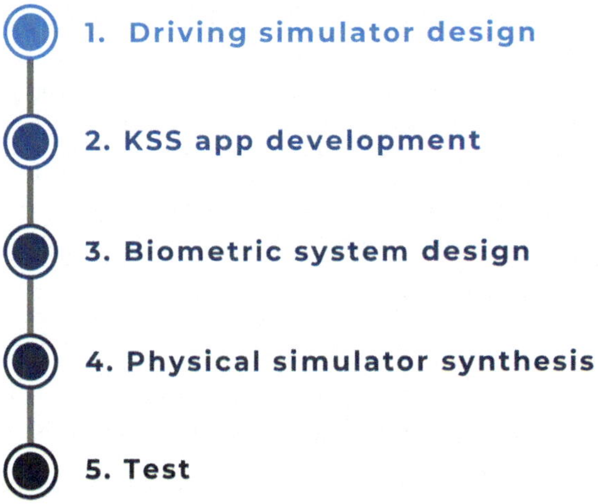
1. Driving simulator design
2. KSS app development
3. Biometric system design
4. Physical simulator synthesis
5. Test

The ultimate goal has always been to create an open-source system with a very versatile structure that could fulfill the needs of those who use it for research purposes. This is to create a free system, usable for different types of tests and customizable according to the specific characteristics of given research activity.

As discussed in the previous section, Unreal Engine was chosen for creating the virtual environment, since this particular game engine is one of the most common software utilized among game developers. The choice was dictated by the level of realism achievable with this tool since the realism of the simulation environment is one of the crucial points for a simulator that aims to recreate the real world [37].

The first idea was to recreate a driving simulator to perform various tests to analyze the driver's psychophysical state by using an existing virtual environment. The fundamental part of creating a driving simulator for measuring drowsiness is the management of the length and configuration of the road tracks. To improve the research process, a driving simulator has been used and tested. Although more specific than a game, the existing simulator presented many limitations. In particular, the software did not allow configuring the characteristic of the driving environment and the road track according to the factors that influence drive drowsiness. The map characteristics inside the software were mainly towns with all their typical characteristics: very frequent stops, traffic lights, and traffic. Not particularly suitable for creating monotonous environments associated with the type of research that had to be carried out. Hence, the need to create our simulator and our map that reflects all the characteristics necessary for the study.

### 3.1.1 System Requirements

The project analyzed many different game simulators that already exist on the market to understand and acquire the fundamental requirements to develop an effective user experience for testing drive drowsiness, in terms of the easiness level of the gameplay and the detail level of graphics quality.

The investigation classified games under three main categories based on their nature of gameplay:

- Open world: Burnout Paradise, Forza Horizon 4, GTA V, Need For Speed: Heath, Test Drive Unlimited 2, The Crew 2;
- Street circuits: AirSim, Carla, City Car Driving, L.A.Noire, Need For Speed: Most Wanted, Saint Row 4;
- Race tracks: F1 202, Gran Turismo 5, Iracing, Nascar heat 5, Project Cars 3, Speed Dreams.

In the end, the benchmarks analysis highlighted the crucial aspects that the expected project should incorporate in the final driving simulator:

- The high level of realism provided by the graphics and physics simulation;
- The general circuit structure that was attributable to that of a real road or highway;
- The layout and a landscape that is less repetitive as possible, so as not to give the idea of being inside a circuit;
- The monotonous general structure;
- Set the game structure to be easily editable;
- Make the simulator easy to use;
- Develop the game free for everyone to use.

### 3.1.2 Requirements Fulfillment

The result of these system requirements is PARIDE, a flexible driving simulator for assessing drive drowsiness created with Unreal Engine. The first beta version of this game features a single circuit of about 200 km in length which can be set up in two main variants: Day-time and Night-time. The layout of the circuit has been designed to get as close as possible to that of a motorway or highway.

Previously we have highlighted the system requirements that were necessary for the development of this project. Now we are going to see how our simulator tries to best respond to these requests:

- This game was created using realistic design assets either found in the Unreal Store or specifically designed to respond to the requests;
- The simulator, even if structured as a race track, has been designed to reflect the characteristics of a monotonous road track such as the motorway, which was equipped with wide roadways, long straights, and very light curves;
- The circuit has been sketched to have a length of about 200 km for a lap time of almost two hours to stress experiencing monotonous environments for long periods;
- The monotonous landscape has been designed to be realistic and diversified as much as is feasible, passing from beaches to mountains without having any particular characteristics;

- The game was entirely created using Unreal Engine 4 (UE4) and all of its assets are integrated into the project and therefore reusable. To maintain the software customizable and open to different testing scenarios, the structure of the road was made with splines and easily editable to be more accessible for other different users with different research intents;
- PARIDE is designed to interface perfectly with any controller, joystick, and steering wheel while the controls are simple and essential to provide an accessible and easy-to-use software to a wider group of users;
- As Epic Games' policy for using UE4 is based on paying a percentage of the proceeds earned from the sale of the games, distributing the simulator as free-to-play is completely feasible.

The peculiarity of the game lies in its game setup. The latter is designed to allow the researchers to freely set up a series of passive factors associated with underload driving conditions that are essential to study driver drowsiness. The first configurable factors are daytime and weather to face the simulation and test of the track at different times of the day and in various critical environmental conditions (see Fig. 2).

## *3.2 The Programming of the Application for the Collection of Data Concerning Drowsiness*

To gather the level of drowsiness perceived by the user during the entire duration of the study, an application was developed for the collection of data relating to the Karolinska Sleepiness Scale (KSS). KSS is a method used to give a numerical value to the subjective level of sleepiness at a particular time during the day. The developed application allows a person to indicate the level of her/his psycho-physical state experienced in the previous ten minutes [40].

The KSS method uses the 9-point Likert and its scale is defined as follows: (9) Extremely sleepy, fighting sleep; (8) Sleepy, some effort to keep alert; (7) Sleepy, but no difficulty remaining awake; (6) Some signs of sleepiness; (5) Neither alert nor sleepy; (4) Rather alert; (3) Alert; (2) Very alert; (1) Extremely alert.

This test was implemented during the measurement to acquire a parameter to assess the effectiveness of the simulator. Since the KSS scale is based on subjective sensations, it was associated with biometric data collection. In this way, it is possible to create a correspondence between the driver sensation, reported through the KSS, and the biometric values gathered during the simulation to outcome with a simulator assessment based on both qualitative and quantitative parameters.

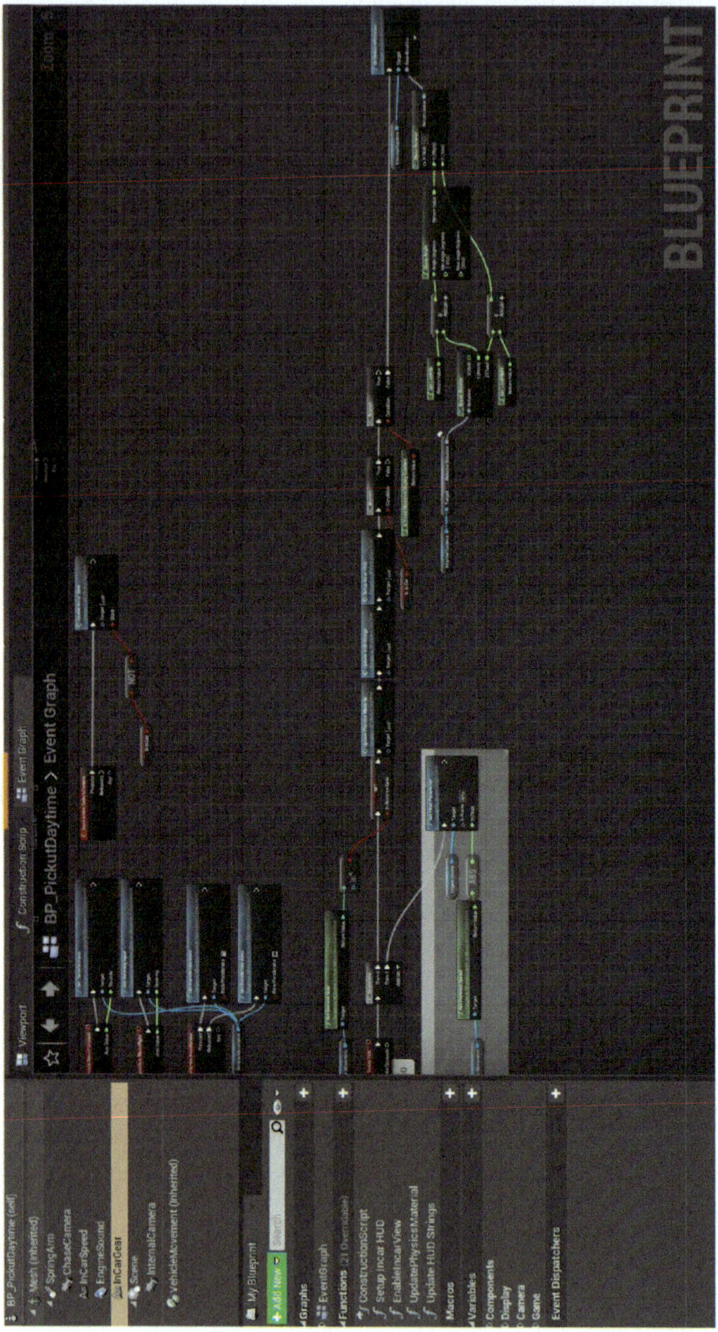


**Fig. 2** PARIDE's blueprint and coding screen on Unreal Engine 4

### 3.3 The Design of a System to Collect and Analyze Users' Biometric Data

As the third step, we integrated into the driving simulator an acquisition system to monitor the driver's status. The device is composed of a microcontroller board and two sensors. The microcontroller board drives and controls the sensors to acquire the physiological signals of the driver. In particular, we exploited the Photoplethysmography technique (PPG), which is an optical technique that allows the monitoring of heart functioning [41].

Since the heart is governed by the Autonomous Nervous System and also controls drowsiness phenomena, PPG monitoring enables drowsiness detection [42]. Driver's physiological signals were acquired on the palm with the sensors placed into the steering wheel.

### 3.4 Creation of the Physical Simulator, the Union of the Three Modules

The workstation to perform the tests has been built within the ASELab laboratory, at the University of Modena and Reggio Emilia, Italy. The station was designed to replicate the cockpit of a car to make the driving experience inside the simulator realistic.

The simulator core consists of three basic components, which are essential to recreate the cockpit of a car: the driver's seat, a steering wheel, and a video projector (Fig. 3). Two other elements were extra added to collect specific data necessary for research:

- The support for mobile devices to keep the tablet with the KSS application stable;
- The sensors on the steering wheel are necessary to detect the data used for the study on drowsiness.

### 3.5 Test Procedure

The workstation served to test the beta version of the driving simulator by running a test for the collection of drowsiness data together with twenty-five participants. The structure of the methodology used for carrying out the study was divided into three main sections:

1. The first introductory phase explained to the user the goals of the research analysis and the procedure by which the test would be conducted.
2. The central phase regarded the running of the experiment. The users entered inside the simulator and had to drive in the virtual environment for 1 h. Every

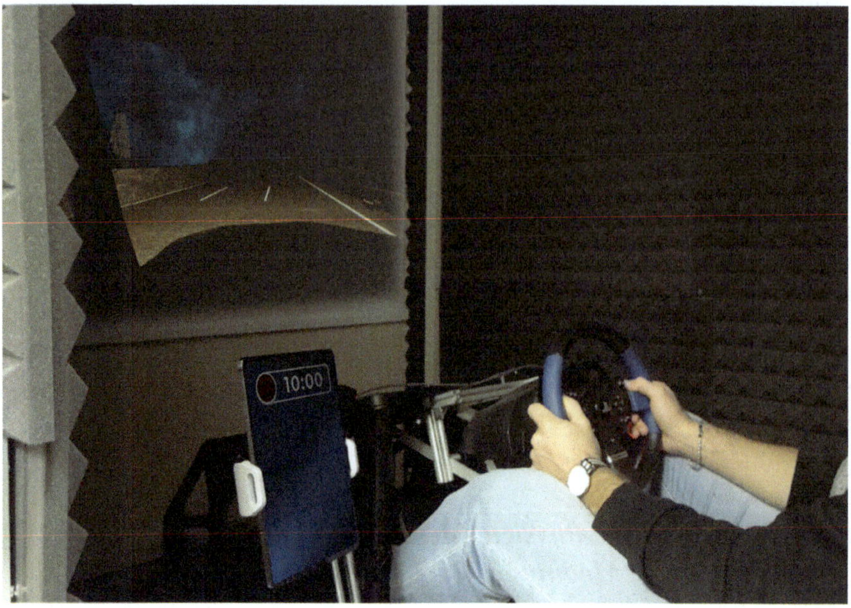


**Fig. 3** The complete workplace with the simulator, steering wheel, and KSS application

10 min the users were asked to select a value of the KSS application. This drive and compile cycle continued until the timer expired. At that point, the simulator turned off while the users were invited to leave the cockpit and move to the final phase.

3. The last phase regarded the assessment of the driving simulator. The users were invited to provide feedback to the researchers. The insights were collected and studied to validate the effectiveness of the driving simulator. The values collected during the simulation are also saved for future analysis during the development and implementation of the software.

### 3.5.1 Three Macro-categories of Evaluation

Collecting data during the last phase of the simulation was used to assess and validate the efficiency of the simulator from the user's perspective to enrich the overall quality of the user experience. The feedback was distributed into three macro-categories according to the area they were going to evaluate:

- The Usability Test was implied to collect feedback and insights on the functional and graphical elements of the virtual environment. The point of these questions was to identify the issues and disturbances associated with the realism of the overall experience of the simulation.
- The NASA-Task Load Index (TLX) is a subjective workload assessment of operators working with various human–machine interface systems [43]. It was implied

to assess the cognitive effort of the users required to interact with the driving simulator.

- The Software Usability Measurement Inventory (SUMI) is a measurement method to assess the quality of software from the end user's point of view [44]. The SUMI was used to measure the user experience of the whole simulation.

# 4 Results

## 4.1 Game Feedback

The procedure used to perform the testing activities allowed the research study to collect feedback and insights on the game through the final assessment phase. The final evaluation of the simulator was conducted through the analysis of the data collection derived from the KSS test and the biometric parameters of the participants, and through the examination of three macro-categories of the final questionnaire.

## 4.2 KSS and Biometric Values

The presented system has the purpose of allowing real data collection about driver status safely. As said before, to validate the system from a physiological point of view, we performed tests on several drivers. Experimental results have underlined a variation in drivers' biometric parameters during simulation. Figure 4 shows the KSS value collected by a driver during the test: it is visible an increasing trend, which means the driver's level of drowsiness increases during simulation. This demonstrates that the presented systems stimulate drowsiness, and also that physiological parameter variations are related to this increase. As a result, the system could be an important and helpful instrument for driver monitoring research, not only for drowsiness but also for everything related to driver psycho-physiological status.

## 4.3 Evaluation of the Questionnaires

The usability test found that the general driving experience was generally positive. However, some feedback highlighted the necessity to adjust the sensitivity at the wheel, the indications for the fork in the road, and the car lights, to improve the realism of the virtual experience. Other considerations referred to the addition of traffic and the automatic variation of the weather conditions as future implementations that can enrich the variability of the virtual environment. Nevertheless, as these last aspects

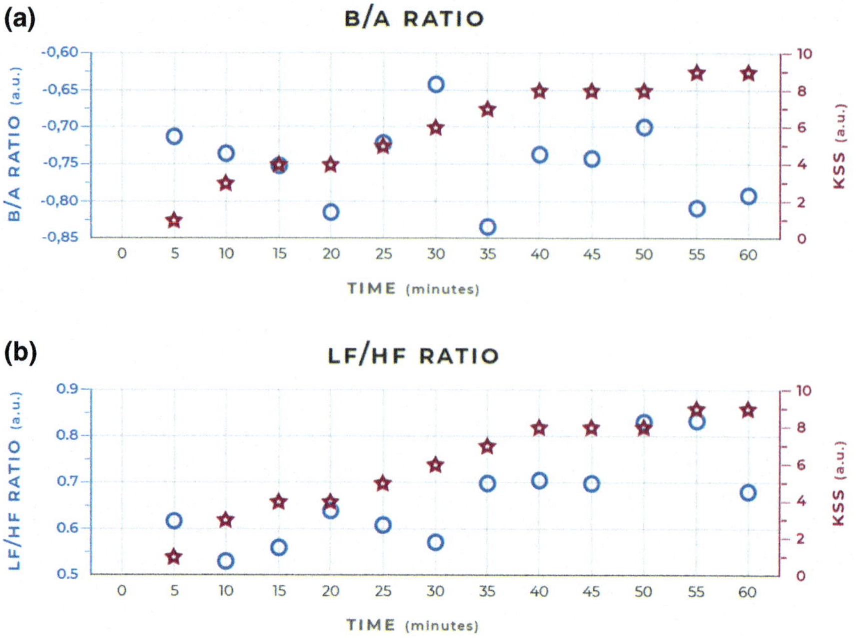


**Fig. 4** KSS data collected from a single test concerning other biometrical data. **a** and **b** represents the variations of the B/A ratio and LF/HF ratio, which are parameters related to Autonomous Nervous System and they are indicators of drowsiness level. The B/A ratio refers to the amplitude ratio between 2 of the four systolic waves (a, b, c, and d) used to monitor arterial blood pressure through a photoplethysmogram (PTG). The LF/HF ratio corresponds to low-frequency (LF) and high-frequency (HF) bands in heart rate variability (HRV)

were already a part of the new implementation of the virtual environment, they were mainly assessed as not debilitating for the initial purpose of the simulation itself.

The TLX test aimed to understand how much effort the use of the game requires within the simulation experience in the six following areas: Mental Demand, Physical Demand, Temporal Demand, Performance, Effort, and Frustration. Those conclusions highlighted the correct functioning of the simulator in terms of reactivity and speed. The simulator in addition has always behaved as expected with no bugs or sudden crashes.

Regarding the SUMI test, the research referred to the experience as a whole, therefore also going to consider the entire duration of the simulation on drowsiness. The simulation, although the same for everyone in technical terms, was subjectively approached by each user. Consequently, the conclusions of the test were slightly different from each other: some users fell asleep while driving and spun, and others ended the experience only worn. Nevertheless, despite this diversification, the test suggested a positive trend that highlights the effectiveness of the driving simulator in stimulating driving fatigue.

### 4.4 Future Works

The results demonstrate that PARIDE presents the fundamental characteristics for the simulation of drowsiness but, potentially, it has the characteristics to be applied and used in a large number of tests related to the driving system and the diagnosis of the driver's psychophysical state.

Considering this, the testing activities reported some aspects related to the driving configuration that can be used to improve the simulator in the next step of this research project:

- Improving the dynamics of time and weather to recreate the transition between night and day autonomously;
- Implementation of other passive factors that influence drowsiness, such as varying the number of other cars or non-player characters to recreate road traffic and congestion, making the driving experience more realistic and configurable for other different driver diagnoses;
- Implementation of advanced physics with the possibility of implementing even accidents and breakdowns of the driver's vehicle and its surroundings to give the possibility to analyze the driver's psychophysical state in different and extreme conditions but also detect better the causes of a specific crash impact;
- Implementation of a series of driving commands, such as gears and other internal settings to stimulate underload driving conditions to the drivers with a complex driving task or auxiliary secondary tasks;
- Adding the choice to select a particular vehicle and customize its performance or driving controls to enlarge the studies on other types of vehicles;
- Adding the capability to create or import other tracks and maps to increase the variety of different contexts in which to perform a driving simulation.

Therefore, other tests are underway to improve the user experience of the simulator as required by the users' assessment. In particular, some improvements are undergoing to make the graphic elements and the advanced physics close to the realism of the real world. In addition, other implementations are addressed to add new game assets reporting the variability of the passive factors that can be easy to configure and use by the researchers for different research purposes.

## 5 Conclusion

Involving the users during the experimentation of the driving simulator allowed the project to test and validate its effectiveness positively in being used for research purposes, specifically for studying drive drowsiness.

Both the data collection analysis of the users and the test feedback gathered from the assessment questionnaire confirmed the validation of the virtual environment. The KSS scale and the biometric parameters highlighted that the more time the users engaged in the simulation and more the level of sleepiness increased. The questionnaire suggested new insights for implementing and improving the parameters associated with the virtual environment.

In conclusion, the first beta version of PARIDE can be considered a scaffold for developing an open virtual environment that can be configurable according to the purpose of other different research studies. The power of the Unreal Engine 4 software permitted it to reproduce a realistic driving environment simulation based on realistic game assets, providing, at the same time, editable software that can be personalized according to the intent of a particular experiment or test.

The introduced simulator is a user-friendly and open-source tool that allows the analysis of the psychophysical state of the driver and could improve the study of this sector. Our final aim was to create an essential tool to gather a significant amount of biometric data that help to assess better the level of drivers' sleepiness. Considering that, the biometric data collection is expected to be used to analyze the health status of the drivers during the simulation and to compare them to understand what are the most significant factors that influence sleepiness. The other next steps will include an AI system in the simulator aiming at processing and assessing the driver's psychophysical state based on the parameters gathered from the driving simulator. This will serve to create prediction and intervention models that will be useful to prevent drowsiness in time.

## References

1. World Health Organization: Global status report on road safety 2018, Geneve (2018)
2. Medina, A.L., Lee, S.E., Wierwille, W.W., Hanowski, R.J.: Relationship between infrastructure, driver error, and critical incidents. In: Proceedings of the Human Factors and Ergonomics Society Annual Meeting, vol. 48, pp. 2075–2079 (2004). https://doi.org/10.1177/154193120404801661
3. Stanton, N.A., Salmon, P.M.: Human error taxonomies applied to driving: a generic driver error taxonomy and its implications for intelligent transport systems. Saf. Sci. **47**, 227–237 (2009). https://doi.org/10.1016/j.ssci.2008.03.006
4. Hills, B.L.: Vision, visibility, and perception in driving. Perception **9**, 183–216 (1980). https://doi.org/10.1068/p090183
5. Endsley M.R.: Toward a theory of situation awareness in dynamic systems. Hum. Factors J. Hum. Factors Ergon. Soc. **37**, 32–64 (1995). https://doi.org/10.1518/001872095779049543
6. Green, M.: "How Long Does It Take to Stop?" Methodological analysis of driver perception-brake times. Transp. Hum. Factors **2**, 195–216 (2000). https://doi.org/10.1207/STHF0203_1
7. Driver, J.: A selective review of selective attention research from the past century. Br. J. Psychol. **92**, 53–78 (2001)
8. Cnossen, F., Meijman, T., Rothengatter, T.: Adaptive strategy changes as a function of task demands: a study of car drivers. Ergonomics **47**, 218–236 (2004). https://doi.org/10.1080/00140130310001629757
9. Patten, C.J., Kircher, A., Östlund, J., Nilsson, L.: Using mobile telephones: cognitive workload and attention resource allocation. Accid. Anal. Prev. **36**, 341–350 (2004). https://doi.org/10.1016/S0001-4575(03)00014-9

10. Harbluk, J.L., Lalande, S.: Performing e-mail tasks while driving: the impact of speech-based tasks on visual detection. In: Driving Assessment 2005: Proceedings of the 3rd International Driving Symposium on Human Factors in Driver Assessment, Training, and Vehicle Design, pp. 311–317. University of Iowa, Iowa (2005). https://doi.org/10.17077/drivingassessment.1178
11. Jordan, P.W., Johnson, G.I.: Exploring mental workload via TLX: the case of operating a car stereo whilst driving. Vis. Veh. **4**, 255–262 (1993)
12. Spence, C., Ho, C.: Multisensory warning signals for event perception and safe driving. Theor. Issues Ergon. Sci. **9**, 523–554 (2008). https://doi.org/10.1080/14639220701816765
13. Damiani, S., Deregibus, E., Andreone, L.: Driver-vehicle interfaces and interaction: where are they going? Eur. Transp. Res. Rev. **1**, 87–96 (2009). https://doi.org/10.1007/s12544-009-0009-2
14. Ho, C., Spence, C.: The Multisensory Driver: Implications for Ergonomic Car Interface Design (Human Factors in Road and Rail). CRC Press, Boca Raton (2008)
15. Ayoub, J., Zhou, F., Bao, S., Yang, X.J.: From manual driving to automated driving. In: Proceedings of the 11th International Conference on Automotive User Interfaces and Interactive Vehicular Applications, pp. 70–90. ACM, New York, NY, USA (2019). https://doi.org/10.1145/3342197.3344529
16. Gibson, Z., Butterfield, J., Marzano, A.: User-centered design criteria in next generation vehicle consoles. Procedia CIRP **55**, 260–265 (2016). https://doi.org/10.1016/j.procir.2016.07.024
17. Pitts, M.J., Skrypchuk, L., Attridge, A., Williams, M.A.: Comparing the user experience of touchscreen technologies in an automotive application. In: Proceedings of the 6th International Conference on Automotive User Interfaces and Interactive Vehicular Applications, pp. 1–8. ACM, New York, NY, USA (2014). https://doi.org/10.1145/2667317.2667418
18. Wintersberger, P., Riener, A., Schartmüller, C., Frison, A.-K., Weigl, K.: Let me finish before I take over. In: Proceedings of the 10th International Conference on Automotive User Interfaces and Interactive Vehicular Applications, pp. 53–65. ACM, New York, NY, USA (2018). https://doi.org/10.1145/3239060.3239085
19. Dukic, T., Hanson, L., Falkmer, T.: Effect of drivers' age and push button locations on visual time off road, steering wheel deviation and safety perception. Ergonomics **49**, 78–92 (2006). https://doi.org/10.1080/00207540500422320
20. Lu, M., Wevers, K., Van Der Heijden, R.: Technical feasibility of advanced driver assistance systems (ADAS) for road traffic safety. Transp. Plan. Technol. **28**, 167–187 (2005). https://doi.org/10.1080/03081060500120282
21. Meschtscherjakov, A., Perterer, N., Trösterer, S., Krischkowsky, A., Tscheligi, M.: The neglected passenger—how collaboration in the car fosters driving experience and safety. In: Meixner, G., Müller, C. (eds.) Automotive User Interfaces, pp. 187–213. Springer, Cham (2017). https://doi.org/10.1007/978-3-319-49448-7_7
22. SAE: Taxonomy and Definitions for Terms Related to On-Road Motor Vehicle Automated Driving Systems (2014). https://doi.org/10.4271/j3016_201401
23. McEvoy, S.P., Stevenson, M.R., Woodward, M.: The prevalence of, and factors associated with, serious crashes involving a distracting activity. Accid. Anal. Prev. **39**, 475–482 (2007). https://doi.org/10.1016/j.aap.2006.09.005
24. Johns, M.W.: A sleep physiologist's view of the drowsy driver. Transp. Res. Part F Traffic Psychol. Behav. **3**, 241–249 (2000). https://doi.org/10.1016/S1369-8478(01)00008-0
25. Soares, S., Ferreira, S., Couto, A.: Driving simulator experiments to study drowsiness: a systematic review. Traffic Inj. Prev. **21**, 29–37 (2020). https://doi.org/10.1080/15389588.2019.1706088
26. Wang, J., Sun, S., Fang, S., Fu, T., Stipancic, J.: Predicting drowsy driving in real-time situations: using an advanced driving simulator, accelerated failure time model, and virtual location-based services. Accid. Anal. Prev. **99**, 321–329 (2017). https://doi.org/10.1016/j.aap.2016.12.014
27. Gielen, J., Aerts, J.-M.: Feature extraction and evaluation for driver drowsiness detection based on thermoregulation. Appl. Sci. **9**, 3555 (2019). https://doi.org/10.3390/app9173555

28. May, J.F., Baldwin, C.L.: Driver fatigue: the importance of identifying causal factors of fatigue when considering detection and countermeasure technologies. Transp. Res. Part F Traffic Psychol. Behav. **12**, 218–224 (2009). https://doi.org/10.1016/j.trf.2008.11.005
29. Waterhouse, J., Fukuda, Y., Morita, T.: Daily rhythms of the sleep-wake cycle. J. Physiol. Anthropol. **31**, 5 (2012). https://doi.org/10.1186/1880-6805-31-5
30. Pack, A.I., Pack, A.M., Rodgman, E., Cucchiara, A., Dinges, D.F., Schwab, C.W.: Characteristics of crashes attributed to the driver having fallen asleep. Accid. Anal. Prev. **27**, 769–775 (1995). https://doi.org/10.1016/0001-4575(95)00034-8
31. Gimeno, P.T., Cerezuela, G.P., Montanes, M.C.: On the concept and measurement of driver drowsiness, fatigue and inattention: implications for countermeasures. Int. J. Veh. Des. **42**, 67 (2006). https://doi.org/10.1504/IJVD.2006.010178
32. Gastaldi, M., Rossi, R., Gecchele, G.: Effects of driver task-related fatigue on driving performance. Procedia Soc. Behav. Sci. **111**, 955–964 (2014). https://doi.org/10.1016/j.sbspro.2014.01.130
33. Ahlström, C., Anund, A., Fors, C., Åkerstedt, T.: The effect of daylight versus darkness on driver sleepiness: a driving simulator study. J. Sleep Res. **27**, e12642 (2018). https://doi.org/10.1111/jsr.12642
34. Du, H., Zhao, X., Zhang, X., Zhang, Y., Rong, J.: Effects of fatigue on driving performance under different roadway geometries: a simulator study. Traffic Inj. Prev. **16**, 468–473 (2015). https://doi.org/10.1080/15389588.2014.971155
35. Ahlström, C., Anund, A., Fors, C., Åkerstedt, T.: Effects of the road environment on the development of driver sleepiness in young male drivers. Accid. Anal. Prev. **112**, 127–134 (2018). https://doi.org/10.1016/j.aap.2018.01.012
36. Morales, J.M., Díaz-Piedra, C., Rieiro, H., Roca-González, J., Romero, S., Catena, A., Fuentes, L.J., Di Stasi, L.L.: Monitoring driver fatigue using a single-channel electroencephalographic device: a validation study by gaze-based, driving performance, and subjective data. Accid. Anal. Prev. **109**, 62–69 (2017). https://doi.org/10.1016/j.aap.2017.09.025
37. Olstam, J.: Simulation of vehicles in a driving simulator using microscopic traffic simulation. In: Transport Simulation, pp. 43–58. EFPL Press (2009). https://doi.org/10.1201/9781439808016-c3
38. Carsten, O., Jamson, A.H.: Driving simulators as research tools in traffic psychology. In: Handbook of Traffic Psychology, pp. 87–96. Elsevier (2011). https://doi.org/10.1016/B978-0-12-381984-0.10007-4
39. Filtness, A.J., Anund, A., Fors, C., Ahlström, C., Åkerstedt, T., Kecklund, G.: Sleep-related eye symptoms and their potential for identifying driver sleepiness. J. Sleep Res. **23**, 568–575 (2014). https://doi.org/10.1111/jsr.12163
40. Shahid, A., Wilkinson, K., Marcu, S., Shapiro, C.M.: Karolinska sleepiness scale (KSS). In: STOP, THAT and One Hundred Other Sleep Scales, pp. 209–210. Springer New York, NY (2011). https://doi.org/10.1007/978-1-4419-9893-4_47
41. Allen, J.: Photoplethysmography and its application in clinical physiological measurement. Physiol. Meas. **28**, R1–R39 (2007). https://doi.org/10.1088/0967-3334/28/3/R01
42. Kurian, D., Johnson Joseph, P.L., Radhakrishnan, K., Balakrishnan, A.A.: Drowsiness detection using photoplethysmography signal. In: 2014 Fourth International Conference on Advances in Computing and Communications, pp. 73–76. IEEE (2014). https://doi.org/10.1109/ICACC.2014.23
43. Cao, A., Chintamani, K.K., Pandya, A.K., Ellis, R.D.: NASA TLX: software for assessing subjective mental workload. Behav. Res. Methods. **41**, 113–117 (2009). https://doi.org/10.3758/BRM.41.1.113
44. Kirakowski, J., Corbett, M.: SUMI: the software usability measurement inventory. Br. J. Educ. Technol. **24**, 210–212 (1993). https://doi.org/10.1111/j.1467-8535.1993.tb00076.x

The manufacturer's authorised representative in the EU is Springer Nature Customer Service Centre GmbH, Europaplatz 3, 69115 Heidelberg, Germany. If you have any concerns regarding our products, please contact ProductSafety@springernature.com

Printed and bound by CPI Group (UK) Ltd, Croydon, CR0 4YY
01/10/2026
02225883-0019